I0100663

Recharge

David Ko

Recharge

Boosting Your Mental Battery,
One Conversation at a Time

Real Talk on Stress

with Rebels 💀, Rappers 🎤,

and Innovators ⚡

Forbes | Books

Copyright © 2025 by David Ko.

All rights reserved. No part of this book may be used or reproduced in any manner whatsoever without prior written consent of the author, except as provided by the United States of America copyright law.

Published by Forbes Books, Charleston, South Carolina.
An imprint of Advantage Media Group.

Forbes Books is a registered trademark, and the Forbes Books colophon is a trademark of Forbes Media, LLC.

Printed in the United States of America.

10 9 8 7 6 5 4 3 2 1

ISBN: 979-8-88750-494-0 (Hardcover)
ISBN: 979-8-88750-495-7 (eBook)

Library of Congress Control Number: 2024923258

Cover and layout design by Matthew Morse.

This custom publication is intended to provide accurate information and the opinions of the author in regard to the subject matter covered. It is sold with the understanding that the publisher, Forbes Books, is not engaged in rendering legal, financial, or professional services of any kind. If legal advice or other expert assistance is required, the reader is advised to seek the services of a competent professional.

Since 1917, Forbes has remained steadfast in its mission to serve as the defining voice of entrepreneurial capitalism. Forbes Books, launched in 2016 through a partnership with Advantage Media, furthers that aim by helping business and thought leaders bring their stories, passion, and knowledge to the forefront in custom books. Opinions expressed by Forbes Books authors are their own. To be considered for publication, please visit **books.Forbes.com**.

To my wife, Jennifer—
Your love and belief in me make anything possible.
I am forever grateful for your unwavering support and encouragement.

To my children, Kayley and Emilie—
You are my driving inspiration to make this world a better place
for everyone. Every step I take is with you in my heart.

To Mom and Dad—
Thank you for the sacrifices you have made. I look forward to having
that honest and vulnerable conversation with you.

Contents

Acknowledgments

This book has been a journey for me. And, as they say, it's the people we meet along the way that make the biggest difference. Thank you Randall, Julie, Delilah, Amelia, Ben, Carl, Rheeda, Ken, Jack, Steve, Aditi, John S., Johnny T., and Randy for the conversations and time you spent with me. The book and I are better for it. I deeply appreciate the professionals who helped me through the writing process, including editors Laura and Erica. You helped me find the words. Thank you, Chris and Lisa, for your strategic work on this book. Thank you, Bennett, for always pushing me to be more honest and open about my personal journey.

Dear Reader

Before we begin our journey together, I want to take a moment to acknowledge that this book touches on some challenging topics. In our conversations about mental health, we'll be discussing issues such as anxiety, depression, substance abuse, eating disorders, and suicide. We'll also explore the impacts of trauma, loss, and the struggles many face with self-worth and identity.

These topics can be difficult and may stir up strong emotions or memories. If at any point you feel overwhelmed, please know it's OK to take a break, to breathe, to step away. Remember, this book is meant to start conversations and offer support, not to replace professional help.

If you find yourself struggling, please reach out to a mental health professional or use the resources listed in the appendix of this book. Your well-being matters, and there is always help available.

Take care of yourself as we embark on this important conversation about recharging our mental batteries.

With care,
David Ko

Foreword

By John "Jack" W. Rowe, MD

The prevalence of mental health problems, predominantly anxiety and depression, has been steadily rising in the United States. This worrisome trend began well before the arrival of COVID-19, though it was certainly boosted by the pandemic. I have faced varied aspects of this problem in different phases of my career. As a physician practicing geriatric medicine, I've seen the enormous impact of mental health issues on my patients and the burnout and stress-related issues in their family caregivers. When I moved on to run one of the country's largest academic medical centers, strategies to mitigate stress and burnout in our frontline providers were a central part of our workforce management, and this was pre-COVID-19!

The frequency with which mental health issues complicated the management of patients with primarily medical problems required that all our clinicians—medical students, residents, nurses, and attending physicians—be fully trained in the recognition and management of these issues. And when I became CEO of one of the largest health insurance companies, I found that, due to their adverse impact on workers' healthcare costs and productivity, mental health issues were near the top of the list of concerns of my customers, mainly large employers who sponsored health benefits for their employees and their families.

This cumulative experience stayed with me after I left Aetna and was a major factor in my joining the board and investing in Rally Health, a start-up with an innovative—and very effective—strategy for enhancing the engagement of individuals with their health benefits, thus increasing recognition of underlying mental health issues and compliance with management. That is where I met David Ko, who describes his personal experience with mental health in the introduction to this book. David saw Rally providing an opportunity for him to apply his very substantial tech expertise to the challenge of patient engagement, and he made very important contributions to the development of tools now used by over a hundred million people. This experience hooked David on the promise, and reality, of tech-enabled mental healthcare, and he went on to cofound Ripple to support caregivers and then to take the helm of Calm, which reaches many millions of people.

Through these experiences, David Ko has developed a broad and deep understanding of the prevalence and impact of issues like anxiety, depression, stress, and burnout, and a nuanced appreciation of the efficacy of various strategies to mitigate these problems, both at the level of the individual as well as a population, such as a workforce. In this book, David articulates the extent of the problem, what he has seen through his lens as a tech-oriented executive-entrepreneur, and what we have learned about what works and what doesn't to mitigate these issues.

This volume will likely be characterized as a "self-help" book. As such, I see it as distinctive. One major category of this genre are books that tell a person's story—with a cancer diagnosis, loss of a loved one, or some other personal tragedy. The lens is deep but narrow, and the guidance offered to readers is often limited to what worked for the author, which might include lifestyle changes, deepening social engagements, or spirituality. These are gripping stories, often heroic, but they are ultimately limited in their relevance to a broader population. The other major category of self-help books includes those written by "experts," most often academics or clinical practitioners such as psychologists. (Full disclosure: I wrote one of these entitled *Successful Aging*.) These texts do not tell personal stories, though there may be some anecdotes here and there. They more prominently present information, based on research evidence or clinical experience, on the nature and scope of an issue and approaches to its management. They are often very helpful, but may also feel a bit "dry," as they lack the personal touch.

The great distinction of this book is David Ko's balance. He presents us with all the striking evidence about the epidemic of mental health issues as well as lots of detailed guidance on what works and what doesn't, but he does so in the context of his own personal journey with mental health challenges as well as interviews with others who have overcome similar problems. This mix of the personal and the academic/ professional yields a remarkably readable and informative volume that can be helpful to not only individuals but also employers and even policymakers. The icing on the cake, which you'll read about shortly, is the innovative "battery" metaphor, which is woven throughout the book and helps tie the various chapters together in a coherent message.

Over the course of my career, I have run two large organizations, each with over forty thousand employees. If I were in one of those positions now, I would make sure every employee had a copy of this book.

—Jack Rowe, MD
New York City, July 2024

Introduction

> The ability to focus and calibrate everything going on inside
> your mind is a skill that can be strengthened over time.
>
> —*LeBron James*

I had my first panic attack when I was fourteen. I remember taking a shower to see if the water would help the tightness in my chest go away. I couldn't breathe, and all I could think about was trying to "power through." I'd had these attacks for a while, and my parents, who were immigrants from Korea, no doubt thought that was the best, most helpful approach. It was the way they were raised. I had a big test at school that day, and I couldn't shake the feeling of impending doom. It took me becoming the CEO of the mental health company Calm decades later to figure out that all those times that I had a test and basically found myself frozen with fear about the looming bad grade I was surely going to get, and having to see the disappointment on my parents' faces, caused me to have an actual panic attack.

But now I work for the most mindful company in the world: Calm. Our mission is to help everyone on every step of their mental health journey. At Calm, I learned about how to recognize and deal with stress. It was only then that I realized what was happening to me when I was fourteen. I've also learned I am not alone. Approximately

11 percent of Americans will have a panic attack this year.[1] (If that includes you, it's not a fun club to belong to, I know.)

However, it was liberating to identify what was happening to me. I could recognize it. I could talk about it because I now had the words. I've learned a lot about mental health since being at the company. Before this, I worked for one of the largest healthcare companies in the world and learned about what it takes to keep populations physically healthy. Mental health was discussed around the edges. When I came to Calm, I discovered it was, and remains, *the* focus. The team works tirelessly to create a product that truly helps people feel better, and I have realized how much I would have benefited from mindfulness and mental fitness if only I had understood more clearly what was happening to me at fourteen.

But I didn't have the vocabulary until now. People didn't talk about their feelings in the 1980s. Especially coming from an immigrant family, we were taught to power through. We didn't have conversations about mental health—we didn't know how. And so, because now I work for one of the world's most mindful companies, gaining the knowledge, vocabulary, and—honestly—the courage to talk about mental health, I decided to write a book to share my journey and some of the conversations I've had with people along the way to guide and encourage all of us to take care of the batteries that run our lives: our brains.

As I wrote, I liked talking about the brain as a battery. It's a simple way to identify where you are and how you are feeling mentally. This concept came up while talking to my friend Brenda about how she checks in with her kids. She had just come back from vacation and shared that she asked her two young sons, "What's your battery level?"

---

1   Cleveland Clinic, "Panic Attacks & Panic Disorder," accessed July 2024, https://my.clevelandclinic.org/health/diseases/4451-panic-attack-panic-disorder.

throughout the trip to gauge whether they had enough energy to continue sightseeing, whether they needed food, or whether they should just call it a day and rest.

Listening to her using the battery level as a simple, relatable way to check in was an *A-HA!* moment for me. She talked about how if their battery was at 80 percent, she knew they were good to keep going. If they were at 50 percent, she needed to think about food or a quick rest. If they said they were at 20 percent, that explained the fussiness she was observing, and she knew it was time to go back to the hotel.

When I asked Brenda how she came about using a battery analogy with the kids, she shared that before, when she asked them how they were doing, they'd always just say "Fine" or "Good" or "OK." (If you are a parent, I bet you can relate. "How was school today?" "Fine.") These bland responses are not helpful and could mean different things to different people—even between the two kids. A "Good" from her oldest was very different from a "Good" from her youngest—and it meant something completely different to her.

I realized that when I talk to people and ask how they are doing or feeling, 99 percent of the time, I, too, get a "Good," "Fine," or "OK" response. And even when I follow up with, "No, seriously, how are you doing?"—people still always respond with "Good," "Fine," or "OK." So inspired by Brenda, I started to ask people how their battery levels were. The replies became a lot more nuanced and the conversations a lot more layered.

People reported everything from being 100 percent fully charged to being completely depleted. Asking the kids to check in on their "battery levels" gave Brenda a much clearer picture of what was going on with her children, both mentally and physically. When I asked my friends and family where their battery levels were, it led to deeper, more meaningful conversations and gave them the space to talk about what was on their minds.

The mind is the ultimate battery. Traditionally, we think of the brain as a supercomputer, able to handle decisions, calculations, and movements in a fraction of a second. But every supercomputer needs an energy source, and the mind's battery frequently gets overlooked. We take it for granted most of the time.

Until now.

The global COVID-19 pandemic made it perfectly clear how important our mental battery was to everyone. As a CEO and business leader, I realized there was no playbook for dealing with the crisis. We all felt very vulnerable. No one knew how this pandemic was going to play out, and in isolation, many of us were staring at our televisions or laptops and phones as we saw death counts rise throughout the United States and across the world.

We were each just one of millions of people all over the planet suffering—not just from the virus, but from the stress, isolation, and fear. Calm saw this firsthand. Our company watched usage jump 100 percent, and even higher for some aspects of the app. Like a trusted friend, people turned to our app in their time of need. Even more poignant, 25 percent of App Store reviews called Calm "lifesaving" during such stressful times. However, while I am personally grateful Calm was there for people during a difficult stretch in all our lives—I also want to help people stay mindful and keep their internal batteries "charged" all the time.

In some ways, the data on usage of the Calm app in times of stress validated a very intentional path I have been on—a path that eventually took a significant left turn toward the intersection of tech and healthcare. After graduating from New York University's Stern School of Business, I headed off to the world of accounting and eventually Wall Street. I worked for Solomon Brothers, which isn't around anymore. My kids make fun of my large collection of Hermès ties, the epitome of investment banking from that high-flying period of my career and the days of Brooks Brothers suits. (I have no place to wear either these days among the T-shirts and hoodies of Silicon Valley!)

I had all the trappings of success—but I was realizing life was not just about money; it was about my *why*, about discovering my purpose. I just hadn't figured it out yet.

Then in 1998, I met Kevin O'Connor and Kevin O'Brien. They were involved with the founding of DoubleClick. I saw the future (spoiler alert: it was the internet), and I wanted to be part of whatever was happening in this new industry.

Even though it meant starting over, in a sense, as a junior executive, after being inspired by the two Kevins, I left Wall Street to enter this Wild West of the burgeoning internet. Eventually, I ran mobile, sports, news, finance, and entertainment for Yahoo!, a pioneer and juggernaut of its time. To set the stage, this was when the internet was not as omnipresent as it is now. In fact, for a time it was easier for my parents to tell people I was still in banking, not "the internet"—because what did that even mean?

The team at Yahoo! was in it together—and we became incredibly close. It felt empowering to be on the cusp of the transformative changes brought about by technology. The atmosphere was engaging and electric, and I keep in touch with many of those great people to this day.

Next, I headed to Zynga, whose motto is "connecting the world through games," starting as chief mobile officer before eventually becoming chief operating officer. What I saw there was that Zynga knew how to build community and engagement among its players better than any gaming company at the time. It also knew how to use its *data* better than anyone else. It was there I learned about the power of data.

But I don't know that I was fulfilled.

From Zynga, I was being recruited for multiple executive positions at Fortune 500 and household-name companies. They were positions of prestige and challenge. But it was more of the same. While they ticked all the boxes, I kept thinking about a conversation in 2013 with another business leader that had me questioning my purpose, my *why*.

About this time, I was introduced to Jack Rowe, former CEO of Aetna, who has been a professor at Harvard Medical School and elsewhere, a geriatrician. (You will read a conversation I had with him for the writing of this book in a later chapter.) He asked me how many people played games on Zynga—at the time, the number was about a hundred million a day.

Jack suggested, "If you reached even 1 percent of those people with something to help them in their lives, maybe something in healthcare, you could do a lot of good in the world." And then he added, "And you would feel a lot better about yourself." This made me pause, and I thought that was an interesting statement, since he did not know me. But maybe these are universal questions: Am I doing something with purpose? Have I found my why? And do I have the courage to pursue it?

It was *another* conversation, though, that jolted me to my decision.

I was meeting with a highly influential and outspoken journalist who was known for asking tough, insightful questions. But I had asked to meet for advice about which path to follow for my new role. Because her default is "journalist mode," she kept digging at me and questioning why I wanted to take the job I thought I wanted. She was relentless, and none of my reasons passed her sniff test. She finally said to me, "Dave, stop being such a good Asian. What do *you* want to do?"

That statement, and her resulting question, stopped me in my tracks. We talked for a while longer about the pressures many first-generation Americans feel, and about her astute observation that I needed to focus on *my* purpose, my *why*, not what the next box to tick was. You know she's a good journalist because it wasn't the question she asked me, but the one she led me to, that I couldn't get out of my head: Was I living to fulfill others' expectations of my career and life, or was I ready to make a different choice?

I realized at my core, I wanted to make the world a better place, which I did not envision being able to do on Wall Street or in the world of gaming, and most certainly not at the new job I was thinking of taking. I had never shared that thought before, that I wanted to make the world better—mostly because I was scared to. So I never really did answer the journalist's question. I thought she would probably roll her eyes and say, "Oh, another one of you that wants to change the world. Not unique, Dave, especially in the Valley." So I kept my thoughts to myself. But at least now, I was listening to the nagging voice in my head.

I left the conversation re-energized. Sometimes we just need to hear wisdom like that to reframe us. Like many people in their midcareers, I had a whole host of responsibilities. Compared to my twenties, when I had "nothing to lose" if I took risks, I now had a wife, children, a mortgage, and a life that I liked very much. But at last, I think I understood my *purpose* was to go someplace where I could make a big difference and impact a great many people.

In this intentional path, I gathered all I had learned from gaming, product, business, and technology and poured it into healthcare when I went to Rally Health. How could technology help us in our health and wellness journey? How could engagement and community—things I had learned at Zynga—work in the healthcare environment? How could data help us be healthier?

Eventually, this intentional journey brought me to Calm, first as an advisor, then as CEO, where we live our purpose.

Every second of every day, someone is using Calm. From Sleep Stories and lullabies, to music for soothing anxiety, to meditations and breathing exercises to help manage stress, people use our app every day. They may use it during times of high stress and anxiety, such as during the pandemic, and then not use it for months—and that's OK. We're there when they need us—and technology allows us to be there.

However, there is so much more to be done—and that needs to start with having conversations about how we can care for our own mental health, and the mental health of our loved ones too. We still don't talk about mental health enough. For some it's cultural (I am a first-generation Korean, and in my upbringing, mental health wasn't discussed; this is something many cultures struggle with—and I talk about it later in the book with actor, director, writer, and comedian Randall Park). Others worry about the stigma, the shame. Some don't know how to begin the conversation.

I was taught to power through my doubts. If I was anxious, I just wasn't trying hard enough. My parents didn't know how to talk about mental health and feared the stigma. It wasn't till decades later that my mother admitted that she suffered mostly in silence in the United States those first years. She didn't yet speak the language, alone with young children while my father was off earning a living. I can only imagine the isolation she must have felt.

That's one of many reasons why I wrote this book. I don't want anyone to feel isolated and alone—I want us *all* to know that mental health and our mind's battery is something we all must nurture and "charge." And I want this book to begin a collective conversation. I've learned so much from experience and conversations with some amazing people that I want to share with you. Whether that's a conversation on work-life balance, or burnout or anxiety, or the pressures of social media, both on our kids and on all of us who see picture-perfect, curated lives being posted, the important thing is that the conversation is happening—openly and compassionately. Just having these conversations plays a part in recharging our batteries.

One of the fun parts of my job has been getting a sneak peek at Calm behind the scenes and meet so many fascinating people. I get to learn their secrets too. Athletes have talked about taking a moment to settle their nerves; musicians have discussed their preconcert mental health warm-ups. All kinds of high-intensity individuals, from the playing field to the boardroom, understand that we need to take care of our mental health in order to operate at our peak. The conversations in this book give you a behind-the-scenes look at how high-achieving, high-intensity people approach mental health.

The people I had conversations with are also passionate about caring for our minds, our health, and each other. I had to share these conversations with you. You never would have guessed that the rebels, rappers, and innovators all believed we needed to recharge and keep our batteries from getting critically low. They offered suggestions and ways to approach the topic—and were open about their own experiences.

It is important for me to say that, even after all these conversations and writing this whole book, I don't have all the answers. I wish I did, but the truth is that no one does. And that's OK. It's my hope to start conversations, to help us "find the words" we all need to discuss our mental health with those we care about. I am awed by their vulnerability—and I feel comfortable saying you probably won't read conversations like this anywhere else. I so appreciate their words and emotions because when we share and have these conversations, we all benefit.

While this book will be applicable for anyone, I have particularly set out to write this for leaders of all kinds—whether you're a leader of your household, running the finely tuned machine of ferrying a van load of three kids to five different sporting events and really needing a clone of yourself, or leading a Fortune 500 company. We increasingly understand the role mental health plays in workplace safety, absenteeism, and the care and support of employees, as well as how we navigate parenthood, leisure time, our partnerships or marriages, and our lives in general.

I also firmly believe that mental health needs to be part of workplace culture (all workplaces, not just the folks behind mental health and wellness companies)—because only then will workplaces thrive. We didn't have a playbook for COVID-19, but we're starting to understand the pressures and realities of work-life balance in ways we did not before. Let's continue to have conversations about how we can make our teams feel better supported.

I am also writing this for parents—because I am in your shoes too. I am in tech—and even I am overwhelmed by what I see my own kids confronting as digital natives. I am also writing this for the "sandwich generation"—those of us with kids at home who are additionally taking care of our elders and parents. I am writing this for those of you who are anxious, burned out, stressed, and overwhelmed. I am writing this for us all.

The battery metaphor is about caring for that inner space inside that we are all supposed to nurture when life has a way of squeezing out our best intentions. It all sounds nice, but in practicality, how am I supposed to prioritize my mental health when my kids have after-school activities, I have a fourth-quarter project due at work, my mother lost her car keys again, and I feel I have no time to eat, let alone exercise or meditate?

As we move through these discussions, look for these icons:

Check Your Battery: These icons indicate a moment for you to pause and ask yourself some simple questions to learn to plug into what your body and mind are telling you, and what the warning signs are when your personal batteries start to run low.

Recharge: These icons indicate "try this" ideas for improving your mental health and self-care, providing you a personal tool kit of battery-recharging suggestions.

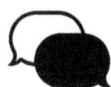

The Conversation: These icons will appear where our conversations offer suggestions for raising mental health discussions within your own family—or in the workplace. (Or questions to ask yourself!)

Finally, before we move on, an important note: In this book, I use the term "mental health" to encompass being mentally healthy—and we address stress, burnout, anxiety, etc. However, this book will not delve into mental health as it relates to, for example, bipolar disorder or post-traumatic stress disorder (PTSD) and other illnesses and challenges that are medically and psychologically complex. I have to pause and acknowledge that there are brave and amazing people dealing with these challenges—family members, coworkers, and even ourselves. There are other writers and leaders who examine those challenges specifically. This book is about how we can all talk about and better care for our mental health on a day-to-day basis.

Additionally, if you are experiencing real distress, please make arrangements to speak to your doctor. But everyone, regardless of where they are in their lives and what they are facing, can join this conversation and learn tools to help them.

In this book, I invite you to have a seat with me when I have conversations with

- actor, producer, and multi-hyphenate Randall Park;
- radio personality and much-loved voice of the airwaves Delilah;
- rapper and Seattle icon Macklemore;
- former CEO of Apple John Sculley;
- former NFL player, Carl Nassib; and
- other experts, leaders, and people who care about this topic just like I do, including my wonderful wife.

These people gave generously of their time—sometimes an hour or more. I've pulled the most powerful excerpts of the conversations to share. As such, we tackle many of the issues confronting us today when it comes to our mental health, such as

- the mind-body connection;
- the science of mental health and stress;
- meditation;
- microstrategies for mental health recharging throughout your day;
- coping skills;
- stress and burnout;
- anxiety;
- our twenty-four-seven lifestyle and techniques to help us recharge; and
- more ...

I want this book to change our national conversation on mental health—to bring it out into the open. The discussion I had with Jack Rowe changed the way I view mental health and changed my life. It definitely made me think—we can make the world a better place. But before we change the world, we have to start with charging our personal batteries to ensure we're at our best.

Let's have a conversation.

Chapter One

Our Batteries Are Depleted

Our World Today

> Faced with stress, too many people feel they have
> nowhere to turn to, that they don't have access to the
> kind of friendships or communities where they can
> easily and openly share their problems and worries.
>
> **—Daisaku Ikeda**

Our world today operates at a hyperkinetic, twenty-four-seven pace with news events—the good, and especially the bad, delivered to us (and the world's children) in real time. Our jobs blur the boundaries between personal and professional lives; there are so many real-life (and digital) pressures on families with work and raising children, not to mention the addition of aging parents for many. Single people may feel lonely. Married people may feel disconnected. We struggle with anxiety, high rates of depression, addiction, and burnout. Certain industries and roles can be particularly stressful, such as first responders or military personnel, medical professionals, teachers—anyone on the front lines of dealing with the public.

I think of Billy Joel's "We Didn't Start the Fire" (sorry, Fall Out Boy, gotta go with the original), with its frantic recitation of world events. It's dizzying. It's almost too much. It *is* too much.

We hear terms like "mental health" and "stress" and "burnout" and have a tendency to use them without paying attention to what they really mean. We might be struggling with anxiety or panic—or those we care about may be. But oftentimes, we plaster on a smile and "power through" (which was my modus operandi for years). We don't have the conversations we should be having. When someone asks, "How are you?" our usual response is "Fine."

We need to change that.

Our Internal Batteries

When I joined Calm, at one of our first all-company meetings, we started with a meditation. We were supposed to close our eyes, but confession: I peeked. Everyone had their eyes closed and were taking a moment to be present with themselves and co-workers. I saw that our team embraced this. The company *lived* it.

While I had been at the intersection of technology and healthcare before, becoming the CEO of Calm made mental health awareness even more personally and professionally important to me. Calm's mission "to support everyone on every step of their mental health journey" is something I helped create and take to heart. Helping people sleep more restfully, manage stress better, and live mindfully is intrinsically motivating to me and everyone at the company. This commitment carries into my "real life" as a friend, a father, a husband, a son, a brother, and one of the 8.1 billion people (and counting) on this planet. The idea for this book really became a spark when I saw my kids and their friends within this twenty-four-seven lifestyle I described earlier. They are growing up in a world, like many generations before them, where everything is moving faster, and everything is a little bit more complicated than it was when their parents were growing up. When they wake up, most of them check their phones first thing—and awaken to a sea of notifications. (Adults are just as guilty of this—we are not setting a great example for the next generation.) Unlike generations before, the pace of their lives is accelerated by social media and the instantaneous ways in which we communicate and magnify events online. The "noise" of background stress has now become a cacophony.

I wondered, How do we have a conversation about our personal and collective mental health that will be heard over that noise? The conversation we need to have has to cut across generations from our kids to our elders. I want the conversation to have a universality to it, and I want to have it with everyone—but more than anything, I want to start this conversation with you, the one reading this book.

We'll get into the science behind recharging the mind's battery with meditation and other mental healthcare practices, but first let me tell you more about why I love using the battery metaphor to talk about our mental health. It gives us a personal, relatable measure of how we are doing. Our batteries—and how we react to their levels of power—are as unique as we are. My 75 percent (a bit burned out) might look very different from *your* 75 percent. One of us might push on through; the other may have to take a mental health day.

It's helpful to think of this in the universally understood context of our phones. We all have these computers in our pocket and—let's be honest—are obsessed with *their* battery levels. Anxiety over your phone dying is real. There's even a name for it: nomophobia (NO MObile PHOne phoBIA). It means "fear of being without your smartphone."[2]

For most of us, it's a force of habit, a muscle memory, to relentlessly check our battery—especially road warriors, parents who are keeping in touch with kids at various activities, busy executives, and so on. We *need* our phones! But I would like to start a new, healthier habit.

If everyone can check in on their mental health whenever they check their phone or laptop battery, we'd all be better off.

It only takes a minute to check in with yourself—but we usually don't give ourselves a second. Heck, I have friends who get to the end of their workday and ask, "Did I remember to have lunch?" (I've done it myself more than once!).

We all thought having these computers in our back pockets would make our lives easier—we could answer emails sitting in our camp chairs on the sidelines of our kids' soccer games, or be more mobile with where and when we could take calls, etc. But what it's done is act like a pair of cyber handcuffs that keep us chained to the office, our schedules, our already too-busy lives. They may also keep us tethered to social media—which can both be relaxing or amusing and infuriating or upsetting. Ultimately, in many ways, our phones stress us more.

Our whole lives—photos, contacts, calendar, social media, apps for our health and wellness, apps to track our finances and help with shopping—are on those devices. And most of us panic when we misplace our phones, and the majority of us even panic when we

---

2   Emma Grey Ellis, "Diagnosing and Dealing with Your Low Battery Anxiety," *Wired,* May 16, 2019, accessed January 7, 2024, https://www.wired.com/story/diagnosing-and-dealing-with-your-low-battery-anxiety/.

see the battery symbol start to deplete. In fact, one survey concluded that 90 percent of us feel anxiety when our phone batteries run low.[3]

It's almost universal—at least in the United States. When you see your phone battery hovering around 20 percent, you start to feel a little bit anxious. If you're in a coffee shop, you'll immediately scan the walls for an outlet, or you'll ask a friend if you can borrow their charger for a bit until your battery looks a bit healthier. I've seen my own kids ask strangers to borrow their chargers! We feel safer, in this world of uncertainty, with that device that can connect us to our loved ones and our online lives, which have become extremely important to most people.

Yet how often do you check your mental health battery, that battery within that is your power source, if we continue the analogy? We don't check in with ourselves nearly enough, if at all. Especially for busy people, mental health and wellness are often afterthoughts—until they become problems—until that battery within is hovering near 5 percent and we're lost in the middle of nowhere and need our GPS and now we're in big trouble. Part of what I hope this book will do is get us all to check in on that internal battery—often. Just like we check our phones.

Check Your Battery

Chances are, you've gotten so used to checking your phone's battery reflexively that you barely even think about it. Train yourself to check in on your internal battery every time you check your phone or computer battery—so you can get in the habit of recharging before your power is at a critical point.

---

3   LG.com, "Low Battery Anxiety," May 17, 2016, accessed November 20, 2023, chrome-extension://efaidn-
     bmnnnibpcajpcglclefindmkaj/https://www.lg.com/us/PDF/press-release/LG_Mobile_Low_Battery_Anxiety_
     Press_Release_FINAL_05_19_2016.pdf.

Before you begin, determine what battery level you're comfortable operating at. For example, I know people who drive twenty miles on their electric vehicles and want to recharge—and I know others for whom it's almost a game to see just how low the battery can get.

For this battery check, just take a baseline "read" of where your battery is at right now and how you feel. Elsewhere, throughout the book, when you see the icon, it's time to take a mental health check-in.

- **At 75 to 100 percent:** When your mental health battery is charged, this does not eliminate stressors in your life. It merely means you have the battery power to handle them. Your focus is fine, you are sleeping normally, and you have your usual level of patience with work, family, and life's inconveniences and problems.

- **At 50 to 75 percent:** You can feel the stress crowding in on the edges. You have too many places to be and too many things to do, and your battery is starting to feel depleted. You may notice you feel overwhelmed; you may find yourself doomscrolling, eating too much, sleeping too much (yet it's not restorative). This is the time to recharge before your battery gets even more depleted. Think about your recharge strategies (or learn new ones in this book—like my Green Space suggestion later in the chapter).

- **At 25 to 50 percent:** Your battery is at less than half its charge. This is when you may feel exhausted, emotional, snappish, or frustrated. You may feel physical symptoms—upset stomachs and headaches, a sore jaw from clenching your teeth, or just run down. "Small" steps to recharge may not help at this point.

- **At 0 to 25 percent:** This is critical. Generally, here, more intensive help is needed, such as therapy or mental health days and other supportive measures. It can be difficult to "recharge" from such a low battery state. Just like with your cell phone, charging will take longer.

• • •

The Price of Modern-Day Stress

The price of our modern-day stress is dire.

Studies have demonstrated that chronic stress "can lead to atrophy of the brain mass and decrease its weight ... these structural changes bring about differences in the response to stress, cognition, and memory."[4]

I can remember people sleeping in their offices during the days of my Wall Street and early internet career. It was a badge of honor— expected, even. We dressed in our fancy suits and climbed into the backs of sleek cars, flying off to this meeting or that one. It was *intense*. And what I *cannot* recall is ever pausing and checking in with myself on how I was doing. Was I OK? How was my mental health? Stress was what I ate for breakfast. And in those days, on Wall Street, that's simply how it was.

I felt that tightness in my chest again. To help power through, I took up smoking. On intense days, I'd step out into the stairwell and smoke, trying to quell that rising sense of doom and anxiety. Instead of "just breathe," I just smoked. I am not sure Wall Street is much different today. (Though I think fewer people smoke. And a side message to my kids—don't *start* smoking!)

Research suggests that chronic stress contributes to a host of physical issues, including high blood pressure and obesity, "both

---

4   Habib Yarybegi et al., "The Impact of Stress on Body Function: A Review," *EXCLI J* 16 (2017):1057–1072, accessed November 25, 2023, doi: 10.17179/excli2017-480.

through direct mechanisms (causing people to eat more) or indirectly (decreasing sleep and exercise)."[5] We even know today that stress makes us age faster. Telomeres, compound structures found at the ends of our chromosomes, are thought to contain the secrets to longevity. Studies have shown that stress can induce damage that "shortens" our telomeres, which increases the risk of developing degenerative diseases earlier in life.[6]

I can remember one CEO I knew prematurely graying. If you want a stark demonstration of the concept that stress ages us, compare the pictures of modern presidents when they entered the office—and when they left. The strain shows.

Stress is no joke.

More than wanting my kids and their generation to care for and prioritize their mental health, more than wanting to have this universal conversation, I think the mission of this book—to prioritize recharging your mind—is urgent, because chronic stress is literally aging us … and sometimes killing us. So why don't more of us do something about it?

Let's Discuss the Stigma

It's hard to talk about how you feel.

Look around you. According to an American Psychological Association study, one in five people in the workplace has a mental health

---

5   Harvard Health Publishing, "Understanding the Stress Response," July 6, 2020, accessed November 15, 2023, https://www.health.harvard.edu/staying-healthy/understanding-the-stress-response.

6   Jue Lin and Elissa Epel, "Ageing Res Rev," author manuscript; available in *PMC* (March 14, 2022). *Published in final edited form as:* "Ageing Res Rev. Jan 2022" 73: 101507, doi: 10.1016/j.arr.2021.101507.

issue.[7] (Maybe yourself.) Consider a company like Amazon, with close to 1.5 million employees.[8] That means 300,000 employees—at one company—are contending in some way with their mental health. But do all 300,000 of them have the resources they need to begin addressing these issues? Have they had conversations with or joined groups of other employees dealing with the same things? Do they even know there are 299,999 other people working closely alongside them who also had to give themselves pep talks to get out of bed in the morning? Have they asked their HR department for help—and do they feel like they can ask for help? Is the HR department even equipped to help? The Mental Health Project reports that 25 percent of people cite stigma and other people finding out about their mental health challenges as the reasons they have not sought help.[9]

The stigma around discussing our mental health adds to the constant cacophony of our twenty-four-seven world. I'm sure we've all heard someone say, "I don't have time for myself; I'm just too busy." And that may feel true—we are all incredibly busy these days. But for many of us, there's also this noise in the backs of our heads, the chorus of our work-first, rest (maybe)-later culture telling us that mental healthcare is for other people—people who have "real" problems, and that to seek help would mean we're weak, that we're "not normal." And sometimes, even if we're not all that aware that it's there, that critical noise can drown out any of the positive talk we might (and should) hear.

---

7   American Psychological Association, "APA Poll Reveals Toxic Workplaces, Other Significant Workplace Mental Health Challenges," July 13, 2023, https://www.apa.org/news/press/releases/2023/07/work-mental-health-challenges.

8   Stock Analysis.com, "Amazon.com, Inc. Profile—Amazon Employees," accessed November 23, 2023, https://stockanalysis.com/stocks/amzn/employees/.

9   Sapien Labs, "Mental Health Has Bigger Challenges than Stigma," Mental Health Million Project 2021, accessed November 12, 2023, chrome-extension://efaidnbmnnnibpcajpcglclefindmkaj/https://mentalstateoftheworld.report/wp-content/uploads/2021/05/Rapid-Report-2021-Help-Seeking.pdf.

What we don't discuss enough is that mental health challenges are just as "normal" as any other medical concern. They can, and do, happen to anyone—everyone. But talking about it is easier said than done. Sometimes we don't have the vocabulary. (Which is why I hope the conversations in this book help to foster dialogue.) Sometimes it's that sense of stigma or embarrassment. However, when we have these conversations with each other, with our friends, with our families, our parents, siblings, kids—when we have the conversation at work, when we simply are honest and assure ourselves and others, "It's OK to not be OK right now," we are all helping to ease that stigma. When we see that people around us, people we admire, are also learning, struggling, and mastering mental health strategies, we know we are not alone. And that transparency is the first step in lessening isolation.

These conversations don't have to be heavy or deep; they can start with a simple question. It's about being open and then *listening* in response.

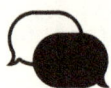

Extending the Conversation: Questions to Ask Ourselves and Others About Our Mind-Body Health

- How are you feeling today?
- How's your internal battery right now?
- Is there anything on your mind you would like to talk about?
- How are you sleeping? (This is a big one!)
- Are you finding joy in the things you usually do?
- How can I help?

• • •

⚡ Recharge Your Battery: Green Space

I'll be completely truthful with you. I do not stretch or sit on a cushion each morning and meditate. My wife, Jen—you will meet her later—is a pretty serious yoga practitioner. Jen can do that. I cannot. But one of the myths I want to dispel in this book is that meditation has to look a certain way.

Here's my own "meditation."

Back in the years of my finance career, my day usually started with bolting out of bed and getting ready to go-go-go all day—and by "day," I mean fourteen hours, minimum. I didn't have a morning meditation routine or even the thought that I should.

Today, and as someone who is so much more mindful than I was during those days, I have a simple morning meditation. I rise and then go outside for just a few minutes—three or four at most (sometimes less). Just that moment of peace outside is enough to ground me in a new day. If you live in an apartment or condo where quickly stepping outside is not possible, even opening the windows is a powerful connection to fresh air and nature. It's something I wish I had made time for earlier in my life. I could have taken those couple of minutes to get fresh air, even in Manhattan, before my day started.

There is science behind this. In fact, according to the Mental Health Foundation, 45 percent of those surveyed said getting out into green space helped them cope at the height of the COVID-19 pandemic.[10] It's not just stress and coping either. Green space and

---

10   Mental Health Foundation, "Mental Health Awareness Week 2021," accessed November 20, 2023, chrome-extension://efaidnbmnnnibpcajpcglclefindmkaj/https://www.mentalhealth.org.uk/sites/default/files/2022-06/MHAW21-Nature-research-report.pdf.

green views have been shown to improve cognitive function in school-children as well as adults.[11]

• • •

The Care and Feeding of Our Internal Battery

World Mental Health Day was first enacted on October 10, 1992. The impetus was to advocate for global mental health education, awareness, and advocacy against the social stigma sometimes associated with mental health. Depending on your age, you may recall that in years past, the topic of mental health was barely mentioned—and certainly not in the workplace. Yet today, "taking a mental health day" is a common expression.

In the United States, we've made it beyond the days where mental health was so stigmatized that you almost never heard about it—not between peers, not in news reports, not in the workplace. Now we see ads from brands and slogans on T-shirts telling us to prioritize our mental health. Which is great—it's a start to the conversation.

Helping someone with their mental health is as easy as asking, "How can I help?" and it comes naturally to many of us. We're happy to ask peers and our families how we can lighten their load.

"Can I pick up the kids from school for you one day this week?"

"Do you want me to handle this report for you? There's a lot on your plate."

"Can I grab you lunch today?"

As parents, mentors, leaders, students, etc.—busy people—we find it easy to fall into the trap of "fixing" and helping all those around

---

11   Kathryn Schertz et al. "Understanding Nature and Its Cognitive Benefits," *Current Directions in Psychological Science* 28, no. 5 (June 24, 2019), accessed January 24, 2024, https://journals.sagepub.com/doi/10.1177/0963721419854100.

us and not asking for help when we ourselves need it. We'll be the first to give you our chargers while our own batteries deplete. The problem is, the next thing we know, we're in the middle of nowhere with our phones about to die and no GPS.

Now I want to share a conversation. I chose to share this one first because *sometimes, our mental health improves simply because we share our stories* and take the time to genuinely connect with each other. *As long as we're open to listening and being honest*, it can be that simple.

A Conversation with Randall Park: On Changing Patterns

Randall Park wears multiple hats as an American actor (you may know him from *Fresh Off the Boat* or from the Marvel Cinematic Universe), comedian, writer, and director. I think of him as a rebel because he is taking a path less traveled in the world of entertainment. I was especially looking forward to our conversation together, because we are both sons of Korean American immigrants, parents who are proud of us—but had imagined a different path for their children as we were growing up. Randall and I had not met before—but we fell into the conversation like we were old friends.

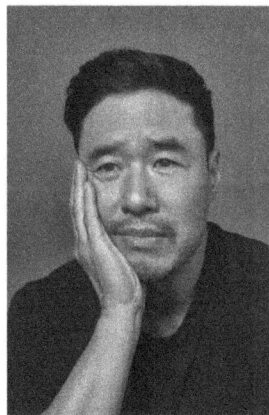

David Ko: My parents, first-generation Koreans, came over in 1971. I recently told them this story that they weren't even aware of. I was giving the NYU commencement speech, at Madison Square Garden, and I told this story of how I didn't get into NYU, and I [just could not imagine disappointing them, so I] had to then go to the school and essentially beg people to let me in, which probably would be borderline harassment today.

Then I was reading on your background, and I noticed this nuance of how you didn't tell your parents about your own acting career. They did not know until they saw you in a commercial … we have that [kind of upbringing] in common.

Randall Park: That was a very specific wave of Korean immigrant. We definitely came up in a very challenging time.

David Ko: Ultimately, our parents really just wanted us to be good and taken care of.

Randall Park: For a while I didn't really get that. I thought they just wanted to shoot down my dreams. But really they just wanted me to do something that would be a little bit more predictable of success.

David Ko: I travel often to South Korea to visit family, and as a company, we work with corporations in Asia, and mental health is newer to the discussions there; it's still a delicate topic. And I was wondering because we're not too far off in age, what types of conversations did you have with your own parents about mental health growing up as a child?

Randall Park: None. It wasn't ever discussed. The assumption was you just have to be strong.

I would see glimpses of the mental health struggles going on with my parents here and there. But I never really thought about it too much. They would go through things and move on, and not talk about it. But many years later my mom would tell me about her own depression after my brother and I were born. About her having a really tough time in this country, feeling alone, while my dad was working most of the time. It was just her stuck in this tiny apartment with these two wild kids.

David Ko: My mom said she struggled with her mental health too; we lived in a small apartment as well.

Randall Park: I would guess there are a lot of mental health struggles in the immigrant experience.

David Ko: Definitely. Looking back, I wish I knew some of the techniques I know now, from being at Calm, on a personal front when I was younger, just about breathing. I had a form of anxiety leading into test taking. I was a horrible test taker. I was taught to just power through it. And now I'm like, "Huh! That's probably not the right way to think about it today." But it was more culturally not wanting to talk through those things that were happening to me.

Randall Park: So, in 2020 during the height of the pandemic, I started experiencing these panic attacks. I had developed a panic disorder where I felt like I couldn't breathe, and I couldn't sleep for two weeks straight. It ended with me in the hospital after blacking out.

I ended up seeking the right help, and then really incorporating this lifestyle of meditating, and after some time I felt back to my old self. Even better, really. And it's kind of ironic that I had this interview with you, because a few days ago it hit me again. I was in a very stressful place, and the panic attacks just hit me.

But this time I had the tools to deal with it. I probably would have canceled this interview if I didn't have these tools. But now I have a protocol, but also that lifestyle change. It's helped tremendously. I was with my mom yesterday, and I was telling her about these recent panic attacks. And her response was, again, you just have to be strong. And I agree. But I think there is great strength in self-care. In knowing when something just isn't right inside, and taking the time to let go of those things and just be present. She thinks I'm too sensitive, and she's right!

. . .

I was moved by my conversation with Randall. Probably because I could see myself in him. But unlike me, Randall was much stronger and honest about his mental health than I had ever been. He is so talented and successful that you might think, *What does he have to be stressed about?* But I know what he has to be stressed about, because I can recognize the generational stress and what carrying it around for all these years will do to you. Compound that by being afraid that your parents are disappointed because you're not following the path they saw for their children. Even if, by all intents and purposes, you're successful beyond what they could dream for you, you never quite shake it. Rebelling and fighting for your true path are not easy.

I was humbled by the reflective moments Randall's conversation gave me. I chose to share this conversation first because sometimes, our mental health improves simply because we share our stories and take the time to genuinely connect with each other. As long as we're open to listening and being honest, it can be that simple. That is the nature of humans—we've been storytellers since the dawn of time, and shared stories make us feel less alone. I also think looking at our families with a fresh eye in light of what we now know about the importance of mental health offers us insights into how we can take care of our own batteries.

Keeping our own minds' batteries charged will not just help us with our mental health—it will help with our physical health, which happens to be our next chapter. I know my panic attacks had to do with my anxieties at the time—but when anxiety or depression or panic comes, it can take your physical health hostage.

This next chapter will examine that mind-body connection and how we can nurture it.

Chapter Two

The Mind and Body

The Connection

> Health is a state of complete physical, mental, and social well-being and not merely the absence of disease or infirmity.
>
> **—World Health Organization**

When I was a kid, I knew the telltale signs that I was having those panic attacks I talked about—even if I did not yet know what they were called. I would feel as if an elephant were sitting on my chest, and my heart pounded so intensely that I was certain everyone around me could hear it. My palms grew sweaty. My breathing was shallow.

But as soon as the test was over, and I got through it, those very strong, powerful physical symptoms subsided like magic. I didn't yet understand that my mind was affecting my body and vice versa.

I mentioned in chapter one that my old "go-to" for handling stress on Wall Street used to be smoking. But I also overate—because if there is one thing New York City has, it's great Chinese takeout at eleven o'clock at night when you're *maybe* just finishing up in the office. (Even better, you can eat it the next day cold for breakfast while checking what the markets in Hong Kong did overnight.)

While the discovery that my suit jackets were too tight because I had put on weight was a clear result of the physical effects of stress (or how I handled it), there are many others, both obvious and subtle. I am willing to bet that every single person reading this book knows the physical manifestations that arise when their mental health is suffering. We'll discuss some of those in more detail in this chapter, but physical symptoms could include

- stomachaches and indigestion (we talk of "butterflies" when we are nervous, of being so stressed we are "sick to our stomach" or nauseous);
- headaches;
- fatigue;
- muscle tension, muscle aches, and pains;
- clenched jaw and teeth grinding;
- insomnia;
- rapid heartbeat, clammy hands, and chest tightness;
- dry mouth and inability to speak;
- frequent illnesses—colds, swollen glands, sore throats, vague feelings of "coming down with something," malaise;
- cold or icy hands;
- forgetfulness.

These are the somewhat immediate manifestations we commonly think of, and you may recognize some of those or have other signs and symptoms. However, as we briefly touched on in chapter one, long-term, ongoing stress can be toxic. In 2007, Yale University established the Yale Stress Center, a mental health clinic established to examine the impact of chronic stress from a multidisciplinary perspective. They cite chronic stress's impacts on diseases like hypertension, heart disease, Type II diabetes, obesity, addictions (alcohol, smoking, prescription drugs, as well as food, internet, or other behavioral addictions), and its impact on mood disorders and anxiety.[12]

Why are the mind and body so intertwined?

Recently, I ended up with an excruciating toothache and needed some dental work done. My battery was at 100 percent. However, when I needed a root canal and was dealing with this pain, it was very difficult for me to concentrate—my mind was far too busy reminding me that I was in pain. My battery drained fast.

And that was a toothache. So many are dealing with chronic illnesses and other physical problems—and still others may have mental health issues like depression (which has a physical component, such as sleep disturbances, and muscle aches and pains), or anxiety (stomachaches, headaches, etc.).

The mind and body are intrinsically linked. It's important that they communicate well with each other—and stay in balance. My hope is that some of the suggestions and insights in this chapter may inspire you to try something new or to deepen a practice you already had.

The Science of the Mind-Body Connection

The answer to why there is a mind-body connection (beyond the fact that our brains reside in our bodies, and they are obviously acquainted) is still evolving as far as the science is concerned. We "get" the connection exists, because we suffer when the two are not in *balance*. But there is more to it.

---

12   Yale Medicine, "Chronic Stress," accessed July 2024, https://www.yalemedicine.org/conditions/ stress-disorder.

To briefly explore the science, we'll touch on a few areas.

The Mind

First, know that the mind-body connection is more than an expression or an abstract concept. A recent study funded in part by the US National Science Foundation demonstrated that the "parts of the brain that control movement are interleaved and connected with networks involved in thinking and planning, and in control of involuntary bodily functions such as blood pressure and heartbeat. The findings represent a literal link of body and mind in the structure of the motor circuits in the brain."[13]

That basically means your thinking brain is intricately connected to the part of your brain that controls your heart, breathing, blood pressure, and even sweating, and more. If your thinking brain is stressing you out, chances are it's also stressing out your breathing, or other aspects of your involuntary nervous system.

Science may finally be "catching up" in the understanding of how the brain and body are linked, but for many of us, this is intuitive. The good news is that if the mind can negatively affect us, we can also *positively affect* our physical health if we learn to take care of our mental health (something we'll explore later in the chapter).

The Body

One of the most exciting areas of research exploring the mind-body connection is in our brain's connection to our gut. We know that the brain directly affects our stomach and our intestines—just thinking of a pizza when you are hungry can make your mouth water.

---

13   US National Science Foundation, "Mind-Body Connection Is Built into the Brain, Study Suggests," May 23, 2023, accessed January 20, 2024, https://new.nsf.gov/news/mind-body-connection-built-brain-study-suggests.

Again, science is catching up to what we know. For example, Johns Hopkins estimates that 15 percent of the US population suffers from irritable bowel syndrome—which is increasingly thought to be at least partially caused by a miscommunication between the brain and the gut.[14] Many people find anxiety and stress exacerbate their stomach and intestinal issues, which makes sense, because science is finding that the connection between the brain and gut goes both ways. Harvard reports that "a troubled intestine can send signals to the brain, just as a troubled brain can send signals to the gut. Therefore, a person's stomach or intestinal distress can be the cause or the product of anxiety, stress, or depression."[15]

In fact, there are five hundred *million* neurons in your digestive tract. The vagus nerve, meanwhile, runs from your brain to your gut (and through many other body parts as well). But perhaps most startling, 90 percent of the serotonin in our bodies is made in the gut.[16] Yes—the hormones that help make us happy.

The Connection

We all need to learn to listen to our batteries, to listen to our "guts" and our bodies as well. Those signs, like chronic headaches or those dreaded panic attacks, are like the canary in the coal mine, letting you know the signals that all is not well.

---

14   Johns Hopkins University, "Irritable Bowel Syndrome," https://www.hopkinsmedicine.org/health/conditions-and-diseases/irritable-bowel-syndrome-ibs#:~:text=IBS%20is%20very%20common%2C%20occurring,during%20childhood%20or%20young%20adulthood.

15   "The Gut-Brain Connection," Harvard Health, July 18, 2023, https://www.health.harvard.edu/diseases-and-conditions/the-gut-brain-connection.

16   Jessica M. Yano et al., "Indigenous Bacteria from the Gut Microbiota Regulate Host Serotonin Biosynthesis," *Cell* 161, no. 2 (April 9, 2015), accessed January 10, 2024, https://www.cell.com/cell/fulltext/S0092-8674(15)00248-2?_returnURL=https%3A%2F%2Flinkinghub.elsevier.com%2Fretrieve%2Fpii%2FS0092867415002482%3Fshowall%3Dtrue.

Most of us have been told when we're nervous about something to "take a deep breath" as a way to calm down. We may notice at times of severe anxiety that our breathing becomes shallower. We can *feel* the connection between our minds and breath.

Science is now starting to support what we intuitively know. Breathing helps synchronize our brains in the areas of emotion and memory.[17] In fact, the author of the nonfiction book *Breathe* has said, "Breathing is massively practical. It's meditation for people who can't meditate."[18]

A Conversation with Amelia O'Relly: The Survivor

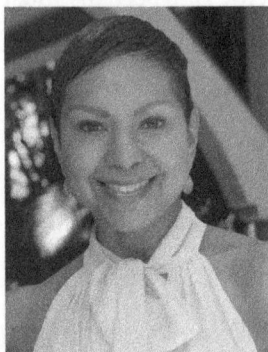

Amelia O'Relly is an inspiration and an innovator. When she was diagnosed with stage 4 breast cancer, she was moved to create "how to Breast cancer" (www. thebreastcancerguide.com), an online site with a mission to unite the voices, stories, knowledge, and advice of cancer patients—to create a new kind of cancer resource. I was struck by her optimism and her bravery. Not only was I interested in her experience with how her mind played a role in her cancer journey but also how she lived through another difficult period with her family's extraordinary escape from Cuba.

---

17   Christina Zelano et al., "Nasal Respirations Entrains Human Limbic Oscillations and Modulates Cognitive Function," *Journal of Neuroscience* 36, no. 49 (December 7, 2016): 12448–12467, https://www.jneurosci.org/content/36/49/12448.

18   Lesley Alderman, "Breathe, Exhale, Repeat: The Benefits of Controlled Breathing," *The New York Times*, November 12, 2019, https://www.nytimes.com/2016/11/09/well/mind/breathe-exhale-repeat-the-benefits-of-controlled-breathing.html.

David Ko: I would love if you could share with readers a little of your incredible background with your family and how you came to the United States as a child.

Amelia O'Relly: My family and I left Cuba in 1980 during the Mariel boatlift. My mother could see how things were deteriorating, and she really wanted for my sister and I to have freedom to have choices, to be able to do the things that we wanted to do. We knew that was not going to be possible in Cuba.

The boatlift was offered to ex–political prisoners (like my father had once been) and their families, but the Cuban government also emptied out all prisons and mental asylums. All [that chaos] descended upon South Florida at the time, and that in and of itself is a longer conversation. But it was just a really difficult thing for us ... we could bring no luggage, no money, and we did not speak English, so it was literally the clothes on our backs. We had to leave everything to the Cuban government, or you couldn't leave. We had a farm and a house, and they seized all of that.

Then we came to the United States, and for me it was a complete shift. When you're nine years old, you are old enough to feel what's happening, but you're not old enough to really understand all of the context of decisions that your parents are making.

David Ko: Those experiences, and the courage needed, had to have impacted your life greatly. Including, no doubt, how you have approached your cancer diagnosis. You've talked about in your previous interviews that you know you remember the exact day you got your diagnosis. Can you share more about that? And some of the events leading up to it?

Amelia O'Relly: What's interesting is the speed in which things happen, so only a couple of weeks before that, I had kind of accidentally found a lump that I didn't think felt right.

And so I started to get things checked, and then I had to go through so many tests. And that was the day when the tests had all lined up to say, in essence, we have found a strand of the cancer, and it's so aggressive that it's already stage 4, which means it has metastasized and gone to other organs beyond the breast.

When we left the doctor's office and got into the car, my sister and partner were wonderful as always. We had plans for that night, and they said to me, "Listen, if you, if you don't want to go to the show tonight, we understand. I said, "This show is happening just this one time, right? This diagnosis that we have just received … this is going to be a while. So I have a choice to either allow it to ruin something, or I can say there are going to be things throughout the next several years because of this diagnosis that I need to still be able to enjoy." And in the moment that's what I decided. I look back on it now, and I think it was the beginning of again that nine-year-old saying, *You have to do this.* You have to move in the right direction and still enjoy things because you don't know what all this other stuff is going to create. So you have to move forward, and my support system became really a small group of core people. That's my infrastructure that helped me get through the day-to-day of something that is almost indescribable.

David Ko: Can you talk about some of the tools and the things that you used to navigate to the emotional burden at that time of your diagnosis and treatment?

Amelia O'Relly: In addition to the things that you get from a medical perspective, I've always been a person of faith. I've also always been a person of gratitude … [meditation] practice has always been part of my life, and that's also how I came to learn about and use the Calm app. It became such an instrumental part of getting my mind to settle down and focus, because there are so many things that are happening at once. When you're going through that, you have to make extremely important decisions as a patient.

I started to lean more on these tools. That and kind of try to see [the illness] in a different light. I relied initially, heavily, on Calm meditation for nausea control, and it was super helpful for me.

You know your hair falls out. Your body starts to have pain; you get neuropathy. You have swelling in your feet, your hands. I mean, there are so many things that are going on, and I was still working. This was also when COVID had begun to take over the world. So the workforce and the human resources teams were responsible for a lot of the work of helping people through that. And I think so much more needs to be illuminated in that space for patients, because there's so much focus on the physical part of the cancer treatment, which is important, but the mental side of it is imperative.

David Ko: Talk a bit about your own site, and "how to Breast cancer." It embodies your own personal journey; as I scroll through it, I can almost hear you talking.

Amelia O'Relly: As I started to feel that I had a little bit more control of my health, I wanted to be able to create something that was practical for people, because so much of what you get as a patient—and it's extraordinarily important—is the scientific stuff. Here's the clinical trial information. Here's the side effects and all that. When I got diagnosed, they gave me a binder with these pamphlets. I thought, *I don't even know what to do with this.* Because I'm an HR professional, I'm accustomed to pamphlets and binders, and still it was so much information. I just wanted to be able to listen to someone or read it from someone who had really gone through it and is going through it and be able to do it at my own pace.

· · ·

Amelia credits her ability to successfully manage her cancer diagnosis to her doctors, treatments, and the mental fortitude from that nine-year-old girl to today. She has gained mindfulness practices—the mind affecting the physical. I am so thrilled to share these conversations because of the story behind the actions. I think of Amelia as a rebel, because of her absolute inability to accept the status quo—binders of pamphlets are not good enough. Amelia wanted to be able to listen or read about the experience of cancer by those who went through it. The incredible generosity of spirit of the people who spoke with me—she and others you will meet—is powerful. I am hoping we all learn to share our stories a little more.

Caring for the Connection

With Amelia's powerful illustration of caring for mental and physical health together, how can we help our mental health by taking care of our physical health—and vice versa? So for example, excellent sleep (and if you are in middle age, like me, restful sleep's probably become a lot more important to you, if only because it's often elusive) will help a body heal and be restored, but it also allows the mind restorative rest as well. Knowing that this connection is real, is backed by science, and can be helped by things like meditation, exercise, and sleep should be encouraging.

As one researcher said:[19]

---

19   Evan M. Gordon et al., "A Somato-Cognitive Action Network Alternates with Effector Regions in Motor Cortex," Nature 617, no. 7960 (April 19, 2023): 351–59, https://doi.org/10.1038/s41586-023-05964-2.

People who meditate say that by calming your body with, say, breathing exercises, you also calm your mind … Those sorts of practices can be really helpful for people with anxiety, for example, but so far, there hasn't been much scientific evidence for how it works. But now we've found a connection. We've found the place where the highly active, goal-oriented "go, go, go" part of your mind connects to the parts of the brain that control breathing and heart rate. If you calm one down, it absolutely should have feedback effects on the other.

So let's have a conversation on balance between body and mind. Balance itself is tricky. Going back to our batteries—for many of us, we're either fully charged, or we're getting low. And then the lower our batteries go, the more stressed we are. (And the more we *realize* our batteries are low, the more stressed we get.)

Check Your Battery: Your Mind-Body Connection

For this battery check, check in on how your mind is treating your body. How does your body react to your mind's stress? It can look different for everyone. Do you lose sleep? Feel tension in your neck or lower back? Does your stomach tie up in knots? Think about how you personally hold onto stress in your body.

After a quick body check of where you are holding onto stress, check in on your mind's battery and how charged it is. How closely are these two things correlated right now?

• • •

There is something to be said for balance, in not living in the place of extremes. For example, later in the book, we will talk about mental health in the workplace. But even as a CEO who is very busy, as I've gotten older, I realize it is OK to not be overscheduled, meaning if I have an hour in my day, I used to feel like I've got to go do something—anything. But now I try to find that balance and take some time to just "be" and not "do."

Many of us had very driven upbringings, constantly on the go for lessons or clubs, a part-time job, etc. Today's parents are often stretched incredibly thin, acting like family CEOs, organizing bustling activity with little downtime. The global pandemic and shifts to remote work often blur the lines more. In a world today of ultracompetitiveness, how do we train ourselves to take a moment to take care of our mind's inner batteries? And how do we train the next generation—who have grown up wired since birth—to find balance too?

In writing this book, I thought about the tsunami of notifications that greets my kids when they wake up and look at their phones (even if I tell them to not do that first thing in the morning). Instead of ten channels on television and heading to Blockbuster on a Friday night, there are thousands of television and streaming channels. Instead of a family telephone line, everyone has their own phone—and that means my kids have access to social media and the good, the bad, and the ugly of the internet all the time. We are bombarded—and balance is something we have to strive toward.

I used to handle stress by smoking, overeating, and drinking a nightly scotch (or two). But what I noticed is those three things conspired to make me feel *more* stressed, unhealthy, and tired. The mind-body connection wasn't nurturing—they were locked in some kind of death spiral together.

Fortunately for me, I met my wife—and smoking was just not attractive or healthy, and in the excitement of our new lives together, it was easy to replace it … with ice cream. That remains a weakness, but it's definitely better than smoking—and I now also understand moderation much better to notice when my body is signaling to me that the stress is piling up.

As for my nightcap—it was *sleep* that made me give it up. Once again, the mind-body connection is clear. Science (and my own experiences) shows that alcohol will relax us and help us fall asleep—but that sleep will be poor quality and, chances are, disrupted.[20]

Instead, I personally have learned to take care of my own mind-body connection with taking minibreaks (these short mental breaks where I might text a friend or just walk outside for two minutes) and with keeping my traveling down to five days per month instead of the nonstop schedule I used to pursue. Instead of getting four hours of sleep a night, I aim for six and a half. I've just learned I am more effective at *everything* I do when I recharge my battery.

The following sections will offer plenty of suggestions, but as you read, consider how *you* recharge to keep your mind-body connection healthy and in balance.

Sleep

During my days in finance, I adopted the very common attitude of "I'll sleep when I'm dead." It's so easy when we are young to pull the all-nighter, to go out with coworkers until the wee hours and show up the next day revved up on caffeine and ready to go.

---

20   Lucy Bryan and Abhinav Singh, "Alcohol and Sleep," May 7, 2024, https://www.sleepfoundation.org/nutrition/alcohol-and-sleep.

If you are a parent, you know that there is a reason sleep deprivation is used as a torture technique. Babies are *big* sleep disrupters. Then we get through those years, and suddenly your little beings have driver's licenses, and you cannot sleep until the last of your kids is in the door at night and safe.

Then middle age hits—and for many, the hormonal fluctuations arrive—and sleep, this thing you took for granted, has become one of *the* most important things for you to be able to *recharge*. And it is elusive. Many of us spend half the night glancing at our phone (more on that in a moment) and calculating, "If I fall asleep now, this is how many hours of sleep I'll get."

If you have sleep issues, you are not alone. Sleep issues from sleep apnea to insomnia affect 50 to 70 *million* Americans.[21]

The reasons for sleep issues range from stress to physical ailments, depression, a diet not conducive to restful sleep (a.k.a., midnight heartburn), and more. Calm is the number-one app used for sleep, though there are others out there that can help with slowing our hamster-wheel minds.

We often hear the term "sleep hygiene." This refers to a set of practices and habits that are supportive to sleeping well on a regular basis—and it can include behavior as well as creating an environment that will help you sleep.

Smart sleep hygiene habits include the following:

- **Keeping a consistent sleep schedule.** This includes weekends.
- **Creating a relaxing bedtime routine.** Parents know that a warm bath, gentle music, soft lights, no electronics, a story, etc., helps soothe young babies and toddlers off to sleep. Adolescents and adults should create their own routines, which

---

21   Eric Suni and Kimberly Truong, "100+ Sleep Statistics," September 26, 2023, https://www.sleepfoundation.org/how-sleep-works/sleep-facts-statistics.

signal to our often-overstimulated brains that it is time to settle down and go to sleep.

- **Creating a relaxing and soothing bedroom environment.** As important as the routine are the place and atmosphere. Even a little blue light or light can disrupt sleep patterns, so a dark room is best—one kept cool. Shut off phones (better yet, keep them in another room or in a drawer). Depending on where you live and background noise, such as those who live in apartment buildings and urban areas, consider a white-noise machine or other noise-canceling devices.

- **Exercising.** According to the medical director for Johns Hopkins Center for Sleep, the evidence is firm—exercise helps us to fall asleep more quickly and to sleep more soundly.[22] However, a vigorous workout too close to bedtime is not advised.

- **Getting sunlight during the day, if possible.** Not good news for readers in Seattle or London! But some sunshine each day is conducive to sleep (and consider sunlamps for seasonal depression or to give you a boost on cloudy days).

Mindfulness

Caring for the mind-body connection can start from a simple place. Baby steps are more than OK if these concepts are new to you. Starting at all is better than not doing anything, and one of the easiest ways to begin can be to start with mindfulness.

Mindfulness begins with being aware. Being in the now. Being in what we ubiquitously hear people call "the present."

---

22 Johns Hopkins Medicine, "Exercising for Better Sleep," accessed July 2024, https://www.hopkinsmedicine.org/health/wellness-and-prevention/exercising-for-better-sleep.

A formal definition of mindfulness is "awareness of one's internal states and surroundings." Mindfulness, as reported by the American Psychological Association, "can help people avoid destructive or automatic habits and responses by learning to observe their thoughts, emotions, and other present-moment experiences without judging or reacting to them."[23]

Every single person reading this book has, at one time or another, been on "autopilot." We get five miles farther down the highway and realize we really weren't paying attention to our driving and the road the way we should. We're on Zoom calls while multitasking, or we zone out when we're tired while our partner or kid or coworker is telling us something. Sometimes, we're simply not all that aware of our environments, much less our internal states and needs. We are all guilty of it—because we're all human.

The good news is that being more present for your mental health doesn't have to be time-consuming or involved—for example, doing *one* task at a time and focusing on it. It might include taking a walk, getting out in green space. You might begin by eating mindfully instead of standing up at the counter and grabbing something while the kids eat. (I was shocked to discover calories consumed while standing at the counter still count. So do "car calories" consumed while driving.) Mindfulness can be as simple as paying attention to your senses when you're out for that walk or focusing on "listening" to where you're carrying stress in your body—and trying to stretch, breathe, or otherwise help lessen that tension.

Mindfulness can also begin with being aware of the *pace* you are keeping. Do you wake up, immediately grab your cell phone to check texts and emails, and then race to your desk after pressing "brew" on

---

23   American Psychological Association Dictionary, "Mindfulness," accessed January 2024, https://dictionary.apa.org/.

the coffee maker, all the while getting stressed over some crisis that has turned up in your inbox? I am definitely trying to cultivate the intentional habit of not starting my day that way.

Admittedly, sometimes the day "flying by" is one of the most fun parts of work—when our team is collaborating well and we're all excited about a project, that is exciting. But we can race through life in a stress blur. Think of it like flying down the highway, not watching your speed—and suddenly you see one of those flashing signs letting you know you're twenty above the speed limit.

Mindfulness begins with slowing down and just being present.

Fewer selfies. More positive behavior change. Be in the moment, enjoying, absorbing, feeling.

Meditation (Even If You Think You Can't Sit Still)

I touched on meditation in chapter one—and that it does not have to look like an hour of chanting on a zafu. Meditation can take many forms—from an athlete listening to music to prepare for a game to someone who does yoga first thing in the morning (like my wife, whom you'll hear from later in this chapter), from formal transcendental meditation to an app full of quick, mindful exercises like Calm. It can range from silent prayer to a moment of gratitude while taking a walk outside and allowing your mind to empty of thoughts for a few moments.

Since we looked at the definition for mindfulness, here's how the American Psychological Association defines meditation: "A state of consciousness to gain insight into oneself and the world." The APA goes on to say, "Traditionally associated with spiritual and religious exercises, meditation is now also used to provide relaxation and relief from stress; treat such symptoms as high blood pressure, pain, and insomnia; and promote overall health and well-being."[24]

Figures on how many of us meditate are a bit difficult to come by. Based on reports from the Centers for Disease Control and Prevention, about 14 percent of Americans meditate at least once a year.[25] But what that figure does not emphasize is that it was a 10 percent gain over ten years.[26] It also, I think, is not a true indicator of just how many of us are meditating, which I will explain in a moment. Americans are figuring out that meditation is beneficial for their mental health—and thus their physical health too. When I think about the four-hundred-million-plus who have used or interacted with Calm in some way, I know that increasingly, people are realizing that meditation and calming one's mind can help our lives.

I also think if you randomly asked people if they meditate, a few would say yes, but that the figure would be much higher than 14 percent if you expand the definition of meditation to include more of the techniques we talked about in this chapter thus far. People think too much of old constructs of meditation, of some image that only monks and yogis can do it "right." Meditation does not have to look a specific way or be done perfectly or according to a set of rules in order for you to experience the health benefits of mindfulness, which can include

24　American Psychological Association Dictionary, "Meditation," accessed January 2024, https://dictionary.apa.org/.

25　Centers for Disease Control and Prevention, "Use of Yoga, Meditation, and Chiropractors Among US Adults Aged 18 and Over," National Center for Health Statistics Data Brief 325, November 2018, accessed January 5, 2024, https://www.cdc.gov/nchs/products/databriefs/db325.htm.

26　Ibid.

- stress reduction, reducing the production of stress hormones, including cortisol;[27]
- improved focus/concentration;
- better sleep;
- reduced anxiety;
- lower blood pressure (the American Heart Association conducted a study with a customized mindfulness program that saw results of not only lowered blood pressure but lowered feelings of stress[28]);
- pain management;
- enhanced feelings of well-being; and
- much more.

If you want to incorporate meditation into your life but aren't sure how to start, there are apps like Calm you can utilize, and guided imagery meditations—which can help newbie meditators who find their minds wandering. Guided imagery meditations are simpler than they sound. The instructor will talk you through a visualization exercise, painting a mental picture of, say, a beach or a park for the listener and helping the mind stay on the meditation. You can also start meditating by simply trying to be fully present in whatever task you are doing—cleaning the house, fixing a car, or cooking a great meal. But just *start*. It's not something you can do "wrong," and with practice, you will see benefits in your mind-body connection, and hopefully your stress levels.

27   Verena Muller, "Hair Samples Show Meditation Reduces Long-Term Stress," October 9, 2021, accessed January 30, 2024, https://neurosciencenews.com/medication-cortisol-stress-19443/.

28   American Heart Association, "Scientific Sessions 2022," accessed January 31, 2024, https://newsroom.heart.org/news/mindfulness-shows-promise-as-an-effective-intervention-to-lower-blood-pressure.

Exercise

Exercise, in general, can help with the mind-body connection and your stress levels (and, as mentioned earlier, can help you sleep better). When I started working at Yahoo!, I still smoked. I had moved from New York City to the Bay Area, where people seemed to be much more health conscious. I wasn't even allowed to smoke on our beautiful campus. So when I felt the stress rising, three other guys and I would trudge to outside the perimeter of the campus, behind the parking lot, and smoke. I remember looking at them one day, smoke hazing in front of each of our faces, when I slowly realized … smoking is a disgusting habit. I also realized that I was getting more out of my walk to the edge of the campus than I was from the cigarettes. I quit cold turkey. Today, I prefer exercising, getting outside, and chatting with a good friend to combat the physical effects of stress.

Exercising—even walking a few days a week—helps to release feel-good hormones for our brains. But it also has positive effects on cardiovascular health, can help prevent osteoporosis, and even lowers the risk of certain cancers. (It has certainly had a more positive impact on my health and lowering my stress than Chinese takeout at midnight.) We all hear about ten thousand steps—and that is great to aim for. But when it comes to our mental health, the most important thing is to get moving. A ten-minute walk after lunch or dinner is a great baby step. Just start.

But in a chapter on the mind-body connection, I wanted to be sure to bring up yoga, tai chi, qigong, and other mind-body forms of exercise and tradition. Yoga's history goes back over three thousand years and is considered a holistic approach to health and mind-body connection. However, a recent *Brain Science* study examined whether mind-body exercise could aid brain plasticity. In the authors' results, they say, "Our synthesis of results revealed that mind–body exercises induced changes in the structure, neural activity, or functional connectivity in various regions of the brain, primarily the PFC, hippocampus/MTL, lateral temporal lobe, insula, and the cingulate cortex, as well as brain networks …"[29] In other words, mind-body connections can literally improve your brainpower—all the more reason to recharge!

While yoga is the most famous practice to Westerners, tai chi is a gentle form of exercise sometimes called meditation in motion. Qigong also coordinates movement and breathing. The main point is whether you try yoga or any of the other forms of mindful movement, it helps your body and brain.

⚡ Recharge: Yoga and Breathwork

I asked my wife, Jen, a certified yoga teacher, for a little perspective on breathwork and yoga as someone who was not always into yoga and meditation (and because if you have a yogi at your disposal while writing a book on mental health, you better take advantage of it!). Here's her story:

> I started out doing yoga from a fitness perspective. I just wanted to get stronger. Honestly, it was originally a fitness thing. There were many aspects of it that I enjoyed in terms of the stretching, the strengthening, etc. I was less about like the meditative aspect of it—I wanted to get a good workout.
>
> I liked certain styles of it more than others. I didn't want to do hot yoga. I didn't want to do yin-yoga. I wanted to do the flowy, Vinyasa-type, and maybe even power yoga

---

29   Xiaoyou Zhang et al., "Effects of Mind-Body Exercise on Brain Structure and Function: A Systematic Review on MRI Studies," *Brain Science* 2, no. 11 (February 2021): 20.

every once in a while. But I could not quiet my mind, so I would be the type to leave before the Shavasana [corpse pose]. I would be the type to cheat on the meditation. I would be that annoying woman in the corner who would be rolling up her mat to leave.

In terms of recharging my battery, I don't know when it was that I decided to focus a little bit more on the ending of the practices, meaning the Shavasana, meaning the meditation, etc. An instructor had talked about how it was the most important part of the practice; it resets your nervous system, everything that you have just done.

Eventually, I turned the corner to try the slowing down and actually doing the Shavasana practice. I was not meditating yet. But it did kind of give me a sneak peek into meditation. So that was the beginning of my yoga journey. Then I started doing it so much at a certain point in time, I trained to become an instructor.

The practice that I do always, whether I'm at the studio or at home, is breathwork. Ocean breathing, or Ujjayi breathing, is that Darth Vader–like breathing, coming from the back of the throat, and I just remember when I started the practice, I thought, "How do you do that right?" It was a difficult thing for me at first, but then I realized, the more that you do it, the easier it gets. And the more present you are. It first calms the nervous system down in the beginning, but then it prepares your body to work. I even do this with our children—it's a helpful way for the whole family to regulate when life gets crazy. It might feel weird at first, but it works, and you can do it anywhere.

If I could share one thing with the readers of this book, it's practice makes progress, not perfection. Yoga or a pose is not the destination. It's the journey.

• • •

One of Calm's most-used features is the Breath Bubble—which offers an animated visual to bring you to awareness of your breath.

Many yoga practitioners (Jen included) use the square breath or box breath. You can try it now; it's a pretty simple exercise that goes a long way toward recharging.

Picture a square in your mind. As you do each of the following steps, imagine traveling along each side of the square until you complete all four sides:

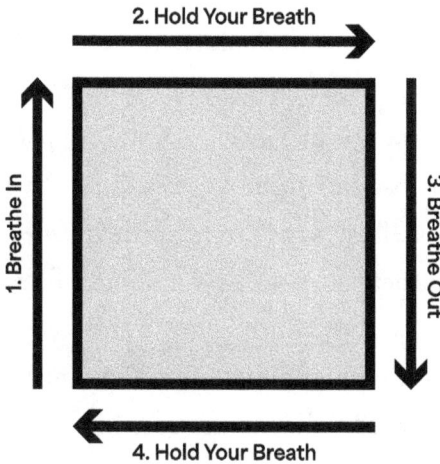

2. Hold Your Breath
1. Breathe In
3. Breathe Out
4. Hold Your Breath

Taking four seconds on each side is about what you might aim for. Remember, it doesn't have to be perfect!

What about the Power of Prayer?

For many people, prayer is a spiritual practice that is especially important to them for taking a moment of gratitude and calming their mind—and hence their body. There are also healing traditions related to prayer across countless spiritual and religious practices, from the practice of laying hands on someone to giving blessings of holy water for the sick and specific prayers and petitions.

For me, church has been a place where I can be still. I tend to sit alone and just "be." Stillness is part of many traditions (it appears seven times in the Christian Bible, as in "be still"). Most houses of worship are places of quiet contemplation, not unlike practicing a form of meditation.

Most people consider the "Big Five" when it comes to religion—Christianity, Judaism, Hinduism, Islam, and Buddhism; however, there are estimates of as many as four thousand religions or more around the globe.[30] As such, prayer has not been extensively studied, since it is personal, experiential, and vastly different across different faiths. The science on prayer's power is inconclusive. However, I don't think science is the point. To the people praying, the "proof" of prayer's power is very much in its ability to bring them comfort or peace when they need it. Their faith is an excellent way to recharge their batteries.

In addition, there are countless millions of people who do not identify with any particular faith but who still feel "spiritual." In fact, a Pew Research study showed that fully 70 percent of Americans feel spiritual, including 22 percent who identify as spiritual—but not religious.[31]

---

30   Mary Fairchild, "How Many Religions Are There in the World?," LearnReligions.com, last updated on June 13, 2024, https://www.learnreligions.com/how-many-religions-are-there-in-the-world-5114658.

31   Becka A. Alper, "Spirituality among Americans," Pew Research Center, December 7, 2023, https://www.pewresearch.org/religion/2023/12/07/spirituality-among-americans/.

When it comes to prayer and its battery-charging power, especially in terms of the mind-body connection, I think what works for you—what works for me—is as unique as our own backgrounds. Radio personality Delilah, whom you will hear from in just a moment, relies on her faith in big and small ways every day, all day. Our conversation was moving and affected me deeply. She lives her faith. There are millions of people like her out there, for whom prayer is a powerful tool for mental health and self-care.

Can Gratitude Help Our Mind and Body?

While I was writing this book, I had an opportunity to sit down with Surgeon General Dr. Vivek H. Murthy. He shared a story about speaking to an audience of high school students. He had them take out their phones. Then he wanted them all to pause a moment and think of someone in their lives they wanted to thank—and compose a text. It could be as simple as thanking a parent or sibling for doing the dishes, or a girlfriend or boyfriend for the kind words of affirmation, or as deep as a note to an influential teacher, mentor, coach, or loved one about what they meant to the person. After waiting a few minutes for everyone to compose their texts, he had them all press send, almost in unison, then hold up their phones with the flashlight on. There was a collective burst of joy and energy in that room in that moment and a sea of light above everyone's heads. Teens and young people, especially because of social media, struggle with self-worth. The surgeon general pointed out how putting that gratitude out into the world is powerful. I found his story poignant because of the importance he has placed on the public health issue of what he terms an epidemic of loneliness.[32]

---

32   Vivek H. Murthy, "Surgeon General: We Have Become a Lonely Nation. It's Time to Fix That," *New York Times*, April 30, 2023, https://www.nytimes.com/2023/04/30/opinion/loneliness-epidemic-america.html.

COVID-19's isolation has shown many people that they don't have as much support as they need—and the problem plagues teens to the elderly and everyone in between.

Those gratitude texts may have made a roomful of students feel great, but the science is there—gratitude helps our mental health. Robert A. Emmons conducted a landmark study on the concept of "counting your blessings."[33] He found, "Gratitude heals, energizes, and changes lives. It is the prism through which we view life in terms of gifts, givers, goodness, and grace."[34] But the science of it showed, for example, reduced blood pressure—actual biological changes.[35]

But, like the power of prayer, gratitude does not need a scientific basis to work in people's lives. It is a way to move through the world that helps us recharge our batteries and face adversity. Every night before I go to bed, I send a note of something I am thankful for to my kids and wife. It's a perfect way to reflect on the day and, like in the exercise with the students and the surgeon general, to do something that makes you and someone else feel good.

All right, a little challenge: Pull out your phone, and text or call someone you are grateful for and let them know it. Something as simple as "I was thinking of you!" can make someone else's day.

The Care and Feeding of Your Body and Brain

I know people who subsisted early in their careers almost entirely on Red Bulls, cigarettes, and takeout at their desks. Or those who worked really hard—but played a lot harder. Most (but not all!) of

---

33   Christina Caron, "Gratitude Really Is Good for You. Here's What the Science Shows," New York Times, June 8, 2023, updated November 20, 2023, https://www.nytimes.com/2023/06/08/well/mind/gratitude-health-benefits.html.

34   ibid.

35   ibid.

us, as we aged, realized the Red Bulls or six espressos or the tacos or multiple beers we had last night were *not* keeping us at our peak battery levels, in either our bodies or our minds. I've learned that occasionally having a drink with friends or dinner out is fine—but after two drinks, I just lose a little of my energy the next day.

Many of us have focused on improving what and how much we eat and drink (when I was a kid, no one told us to "hydrate" unless it was drinking from the garden hose on a hot day outside bike riding or playing). But I also know it's tempting to fall back on old habits in times of stress. When we're trying to crush a deadline, it's easy to eliminate sleep in favor of more caffeine.

However, the reality is healthy nutrition is essential for our mind-body connection. Earlier in the book, I wrote that our guts make 90 percent of our serotonin—which helps us with sleep, moods, and even inhibition of pain. In order to make serotonin, our digestive tract needs "good" bacteria—which guard against inflammation and help that gut-brain connection.

We have all heard the phrase "You are what you eat." I know when I gave up Chinese takeout in favor of cleaner eating, I felt better. But it goes deeper than that. Per Harvard Medical School:[36]

Studies have compared "traditional" diets, like the Mediterranean and the traditional Japanese diet, to a typical "Western" diet and have found that the risk of depression is 25 percent to 35 percent lower in those who eat a traditional diet. Scientists account for this difference because these traditional diets tend to be high in vegetables, fruits, unprocessed grains, and fish and seafood, and to contain only modest amounts of lean meats and dairy. They are also void of processed and

---

36   Eva Selhub, "Nutritional Psychiatry: Your Brain on Food," *Harvard Health Publishing,* September 18, 2022, accessed January 23, 2024, https://www.health.harvard.edu/blog/nutritional-psychiatry-your-brain-on-food-201511168626 .

refined foods and sugars, which are staples of the "Western" dietary pattern. In addition, many of these unprocessed foods are fermented, and therefore act as natural probiotics.

Look, this isn't a diet book, and you don't need me nagging you on what to eat (especially since I do like my ice cream). There are enough books and doctors and articles on healthy eating. But if you are starting to take the importance of recharging your mental battery more seriously, consider how you can nurture it, even if you start with baby steps when it comes to mindful eating. For example, I know someone with anxiety who gave up coffee for tea. Caffeine is a stimulant—and some people are more sensitive to it than others.[37] The important thing is to apply the same mindfulness you are hopefully starting to apply in your life to mindful choices of feeding your body—and mind—as best you can.

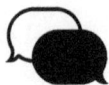

Extending the Conversation: Questions to Ask Ourselves and Others About Our Mind-Body Health

- When was the last time today that you paused to breathe?
- How is the "balance" in your life? If you say, "What balance?" what steps can you take to nurture your mental and physical health right now?
- How are you sleeping? Do you wake refreshed?
- What's keeping you up at nights? Keep a light journal to see if any patterns emerge and adjust your behavior. That's how I discovered that I should cut down on my drinking.

---

37 Hannah Singleton, "What to Do if Caffeine Makes You Anxious," New York Times, June 3, 2024, updated June 10, 2024, https://www.nytimes.com/2024/06/03/well/mind/caffeine-anxiety.html.

- What was the last thing you ate today? How did you feel afterward?
- Where in your body do you notice the effects when your mental health is not where it should be?
- How much caffeine are you using to get through the day—and do you feel it might be causing anxiousness?

Recharge Your Battery: Be Present

Here are four simple mindfulness techniques you can try:

1. **Eat mindfully.** Intentionally eat more slowly, paying attention to your food, not multitasking. Put your phone away for your meal.
2. **Take minibreaks.** I set an alarm on my phone a dozen or more times a day to remind me to take a minibreak. I might take a short walk outside or call or text a friend to say hi. Honestly, sometimes I just sit for a minute to press pause on the dizzying pace of work.
3. **Meditate for one-minute.** Just sixty seconds—which can honestly feel much longer sometimes and can be more restorative than you think a minute might be. Try it now.
4. **Practice deep breathing.** Take two minutes to breathe deeply and to concentrate on your breath. Set an alarm to do it later today.

A Conversation with Delilah: On Living with Purpose

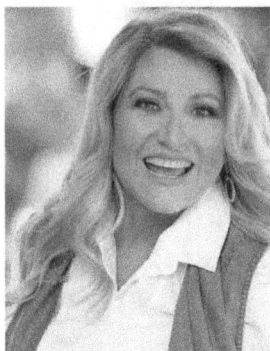

Delilah is an American radio personality, author, and philanthropist, best known for her nationally syndicated nightly radio program that features personal stories, song requests, and dedications. Her unique mix of compassionate listening, storytelling, and encouragement has made her the most-listened-to woman on radio, with more than eight million listeners tuning in each month across the United States and internationally via the Armed Forces Network. She also reaches audiences through her iHeartRadio channel and her podcasts, "Love Someone with Delilah" and "Hey, It's Delilah."

Delilah has been honored with the Marconi Award and inducted into both the National Association of Broadcasters (NAB) Broadcasting Hall of Fame and the National Radio Hall of Fame.

Delilah's personal journey as a wife and mother to biological, foster, and adopted children, as well as stepchildren, resonates deeply with listeners. She has experienced great joys and profound loss, including the deaths of her sons Sammy, Zack, and Ryan. Despite these tragedies, Delilah has found strength through prayer and gratitude, which she shared in a meaningful conversation about how these practices have helped her define her purpose.

This conversation with her was especially meaningful because—transcending mind and body—Delilah shared how prayer and gratitude have helped her find her purpose. I think of her as one of the rebels in this book, doing radio her own way with a positive spin.

David Ko: Talk to me a little about these two questions you say altered your life. I think readers will gain insight from this part of your story.

Delilah: This changed the trajectory of my life, changed me on a cellular level. Pastor Mike, my first Pastor, said that he believes there are only going to be two questions that I am asked when I leave this earth and leave my body behind. Number one: What did you do with me [God]? Did you know me? Did you include me?

Did you use your religion as a way to manipulate and hurt others? Or did you have a personal, meaningful relationship with me?

And number two, he said, is, What did you do with every person that I placed in your path? Did you love them?

David Ko: That definitely makes you stop and think.

Delilah: And I raised my hand, and I'm like, "Pastor Mike, you don't mean, like, every person. You're just talking about, you know, like your spouse, your significant other, your kids." He goes: "No. I believe God is going to hold us accountable for our interactions with every person he placed in our path. Were we kind? Did we show love? And no, there's not a category of people that you get to dismiss because they annoy you. There's not a group of people that you get to not only dismiss but dislike because they wounded you. What did you do with every person I placed in your path?

"Did you love them?"

And when you frame your day—you know, I'm an artist, and so love finding antique frames to put my artwork in. When you frame the content of your life around those two questions, everything changes.

It's not about how many likes you get or how many hearts you get. It's not about how many zeros there are in your bank account. It's not about how many PhDs or letters are after your name, or before your name, or awards you've got hanging on your wall.

How did you treat every person God placed in your life?

If I could do one thing in my life, I would pose that question to everybody, and ask them to build their life on that concept that every person you meet is on purpose. Every single human being. And for me, because I love animals, every living creature that I encounter, I believe is on purpose.

How do I honor their "on purposeness"? How do I honor their being?

Am I kind? Am I patient? Am I understanding? Do I look beyond the surface and take the time to go, "Wow! What led you to this place?"

There's a young man in our community who has mental illness and drug addiction, and somebody posted a picture of him on our community page, saying he was acting sketchy outside their house, and just comment after comment after comment was ugly [even threatening violence]. *Did you call the cops? He looks like a freak.* I'm reading these, and I'm crying, and I'm praying for this kid. And halfway down somebody said, "That's my nephew. He's on the autism spectrum. He's been bullied his whole life. Can you please be kind?"

Everybody you meet is somebody's nephew. Somebody's child. Somebody's mom or dad, somebody's sister.

David Ko: Powerful, that idea of purpose … and kindness.

Delilah: We're on purpose. I don't care what your faith is. If you're breathing. If you have a heartbeat, you are here on purpose.

David Ko: People who have reported having a higher sense of purpose tend to experience higher levels of what you call satisfaction, or happiness, or overall well-being. It's even been linked to improving physical health.[38] Now, given your work with kids, how do you take care of your mental health, so you can be more purposeful with others?

Delilah: I think just like my relationship with the Almighty has to be a part of who I am, not a destination or an appointment, the same with mental health. Especially if I am not doing the things that I need to do to take care of me—and I don't mean in a selfish way, I mean in a practical, daily way. There are times I need to be alone. It doesn't happen very often, but I'll go get in the car, and my kids will be like, "Can I go to the store with you?" And I will respond, "No, Mama needs a few minutes right now," and I will drive to the back of my property. And sometimes I will just have a good cry in my car, [for] whatever is on my heart that I need to weep over. I don't want to put it on the kids. I don't want them to say, "What's wrong? What did I do?" But I need to do that for me.

I also take Saturday off as a Sabbath. I don't work. I don't answer emails. I just spend time with my kids.

David Ko: As a parent, a father, I do want to express my condolences for your losses. And if you're comfortable, sharing a little bit more about Sammy, Ryan, and Zack. You had mentioned that a grief counselor was the best thing you did for yourself. Can you just talk a little bit more about that experience?

Delilah: I did not see a grief counselor after we lost Sammy in 2012, and I wish that I had in hindsight. But when we lost Zack, a friend of mine had lost her son the year before to suicide, and she came to me and said, "Here's a phone number. I want you to call this person. I want you to reach out. I know you have your faith. I know you have

---

38   Heidi Godman, "10 Ways to Find Purpose in Life," November 1, 2023, https://www.health.harvard.edu/mind-and-mood/10-ways-to-find-purpose-in-life.

your family, but you need somebody that you can talk to where you don't have to worry about how it's going to impact them."

And that was a gift I gave myself, and my husband is actually right now looking for a counselor. It's been a couple of years since we lost my stepson, but he thought he should be able to get over it. I said, "Honey, you're never going to get over it. We don't get over these things, but we can learn to live around it."

You can learn to live around the hole in your heart.

• • •

Each of us has a hole in our heart—it may be from a different trauma, a different grief from Delilah's, a pain unique to us, but we each have something—a sacred space we hold in our heart for the losses we have suffered. Imagine if more of us felt comfortable talking about this, if we all had Delilah's courage? Fear and shame often hold us back. Not Delilah—another rebel. It is my hope the conversations in this book can start to normalize vulnerability, as well as remind us that recognizing the holes in our hearts and caring for our mental health is a necessity.

Delilah spoke so movingly about loss and love that it made me think even more about my role as a leader in helping to normalize mental health discussions. I want my team to know mental health is a priority. Our next chapter looks at mental health issues where we work—and how to recharge in the workplace.

Chapter Three

Mental Health and the Workplace

Caring for Ourselves and Our Colleagues

> How is everybody doing?
>
> **—Elmo**

I don't think we're OK.

When the Sesame Street character Elmo put out a simple question on X, formerly Twitter, the furry red guy could not have predicted nearly 180 million views within days.[39] The thousands and thousands of responses ranged from the humorous to the lonely, the sad and the isolated. This one question, posed by America's favorite puppet, started a national conversation. The message read: "Elmo is just checking in! How is everybody doing?"

---

39   Bill Chappell, "Elmo Takes a Turn as a Therapist after Asking, 'How Is Everybody doing?'" NPR, January 31, 2024, https://www.npr.org/2024/01/31/1228145269/elmo-therapist-asking-how-is-everybody-doing.

Answers ranged from: "Elmo each day the abyss we stare into grows a unique horror. One that was previously unfathomable in nature. Our inevitable doom which once accelerated in years, or months, now accelerates in hours, even minutes. However I did have a good grapefruit earlier, thank you for asking"[40] to "Elmo sorry but this above Elmo's pay grade."[41] But in the end, Elmo said he was glad he asked.

We are not OK. Especially in this postpandemic world, the US surgeon general called our current mental health crisis the defining public health crisis of our time. The Office of the Surgeon General has also released their first report on workplace mental health, spotlighting the foundational role companies play in protecting mental health.[42] The report states, "The COVID-19 pandemic brought the relationship between work and well-being into clearer focus"[43] and provides the following stats:

- 76 percent of US workers reported at least one symptom of a mental health condition.
- 84 percent said workplace conditions had contributed to at least one mental health challenge.
- 81 percent of workers said they will look for workplaces that support mental health in the future.[44]

---

40   A. J. Willingham, "Elmo Asked People Online How They Were Doing. He Got an Earful," CNN, January 31, 2024, https://www.cnn.com/2024/01/31/health/elmo-checking-in-x-wellness-cec/index.html.

41   Ibid.

42   Garen Staglin, "CEO Required Reading: US Surgeon General Framework on Workplace Mental Health," Forbes, November 21, 2022, https://www.forbes.com/sites/onemind/2022/11/21/ceo-required-reading-us-surgeon-general-framework-on-workplace-mental-health/?sh=4f8859f27131.

43   US Department of Health and Human Services, "Workplace Mental Health & Well-Being," accessed July 2024, https://www.hhs.gov/surgeongeneral/priorities/workplace-well-being/index.html.

44   Ibid.

More and more employees are asking for mental health support from their organizations, but what does that look like in practice? According to the American Psychological Association, there are four key support systems the majority of employees seek (Figure 3.1):[45]

Percentage of workers who want the following mental health supports from their employer:

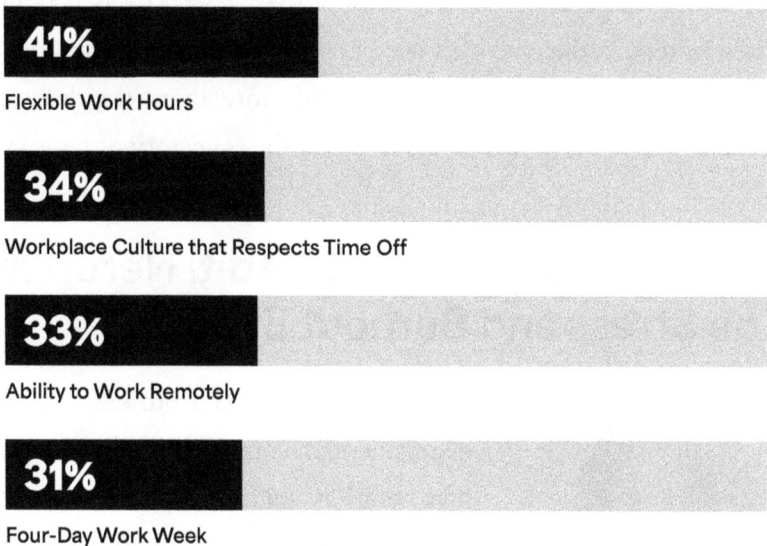

41%

Flexible Work Hours

34%

Workplace Culture that Respects Time Off

33%

Ability to Work Remotely

31%

Four-Day Work Week

Figure 3.1: Mental health supports employees seek (American Psychological Association)

Spotlighting the role of mental health in the workplace, the US surgeon general posited that long working hours, limited autonomy, and low wages aren't just driving a US labor shortage but may actually

---

45   American Psychological Association, "Workers Appreciate and Seek Mental Health Support in the Workplace," accessed July 2024, https://www.apa.org/pubs/reports/work-well-being/2022-mental-health-support.

be at the heart of the nation's mental health crisis.[46] Our country—and the world, really—saw record levels of burnout during the pandemic.[47]

In one journal article on healthcare workers during the pandemic, "data from more than 7,000 professionals found that the prevalence of PTSD symptoms and anxiety and depression ranged from 9.6 percent to 51 percent and 20 percent to 75 percent, respectively."[48]

While the stress healthcare professionals face is acute, stress is prevalent in every workplace around the globe—even at Calm. What we have to unpack is: What is causing the stress? And is it healthy stress, or toxic resilience? This was part of what my conversation with Dr. Aditi Nerurkar covered, who shared more about the difference between the two and how stress changed the trajectory of her career.

A Conversation with Dr. Aditi Nerurkar: The Stress and Burnout Expert

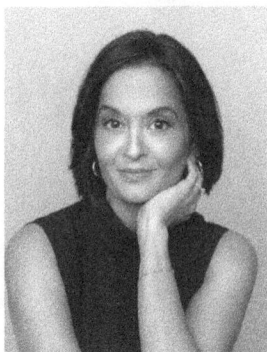

I sat down to talk to a professional who experienced the stress of frontline workers first-hand: Dr. Aditi Nerurkar. She wrote the book *The 5 Resets: Rewire Your Brain and Body for Less Stress and More Resilience*. A Harvard stress expert, MD, TV correspondent, and more, she helped me dive deeper into the topic of stress and burnout—in and outside the workplace.

---

46 US Department of Health and Human Services, "Workplace Mental Health & Well-Being."

47 Ashley Abramson, "Burnout and Stress Are Everywhere," American Psychological Association 2022 *Trends Report* 53, no. 1 (January 1, 2022): 72, https://www.apa.org/monitor/2022/01/special-burnout-stress.

48 Cristina Lluch et al., "The Impact of the COVID-19 Pandemic on Burnout, Compassion Fatigue, and Compassion Satisfaction in Healthcare Personnel: A Systematic Review of the Literature Published during the First Year of the Pandemic," Healthcare 10, no. 2 (February 13, 2022): 364, https://doi.org/10.3390/healthcare10020364.

Aditi Nerurkar: My journey to becoming a doctor with an expertise in stress, burnout, resilience, and mental health began when I was a medical trainee who surprisingly became a stressed patient with unexplainable symptoms. I was working eighty hours a week in a wonderful, but rigorous, training program as a medical resident in a city, then-known as the "most dangerous" in America.

During my long hours at the hospital, I saw things that no layperson should see, the types of crises that you'd expect in combat or in a war-torn area, such as pregnant bellies with bullet wounds. At the time the lexicon of words like stress, burn-out, and self-care, were unheard of as a mental health considerations in the environment of a very busy hospital, David.

And I remember this day like it was yesterday. I was a first-year medical student, seated in an auditorium filled with my peers. One of our professors stood in the front and said, "You know, pressure makes diamonds, and you are all diamonds in the making."

From that day forward, anytime I faced difficulties or challenges, I would think, "Hey, diamond in the making here."

And then my diamond started to crack.

It began in my second year of residency. I was the doctor in charge of the cardiac ICU. I was taking care of everyone else's hearts, and paying no attention to my own. When you're a medical resident, you're always on the go at the hospital, which means you eat erratic meals, and get very little sleep. It's a medical trainee badge of honor. You think, "I'm resilient. I can handle everything, I'm a hard worker," and you pride yourself on all these things that are turning you into a "diamond."

My stress symptoms came on suddenly. I was just rounding on my patients and I developed palpitations. It felt like a stampede of wild horses across my chest, and I immediately sat down. The nurse who I was working with brought me some orange juice, and we laughed it off as lack of sleep and low blood sugar.

But every night, after working these overnight shifts, I would get that stampede of wild horses again, right when my head hit the pillow to sleep. It happened night after night for two weeks. I finally decided to see a doctor who ordered a full medical workup. It was the million dollar workup: heart ultrasound (echocardiogram), EKG, blood tests, everything. When the results came in, I was told with a big smile, "Everything is great. You're normal. Every test came back fine. It's just stress. We've all been there. Try to relax."

So I did. I went out with friends. I watched movies, I had great dinners out. I went to a spa, some retail therapy, and spent time with family and friends. Nothing changed the nightly palpitations.

My initial reaction when they said, "It's just stress" was "It can't be. Stress doesn't happen to people like me. I'm resilient. I'm a diamond in the making."

When they found no medical reasons for my palpitations, I put on my own scientist hat and started digging into the science of what was going on with me. I looked into the science of stress and burnout and the impact on the brain and body. And I found my own way out through meditation and yoga, at first. I learned deep breathing in my first-ever yoga class, and that night the stampede of wild horses became like a trot of ponies.

It wasn't as severe, and over the course of several weeks—nothing is a magic bullet—slowly the palpitations dissipated. When I made my way out of that dark tunnel of stress, I said, I want to be the doctor that I needed during that difficult time. And then that's what I decided to do.

David Ko: That's a powerful story. Let's unpack that for a moment, and let me ask you, for the readers of this book: What is stress, and what are some of the misconceptions around it? What do you think we need to know about it?

Aditi Nerurkar: Not all stress is created equal. There is good stress and bad stress. The misconception is that all stress is bad, and that's not true, scientifically. There is such a thing as healthy stress—we call this adaptive stress. Everything good in all our lives was created because of a little bit of healthy stress. Getting a degree from high school, vocational school, or college, finding your first job, maybe buying your first car, moving in with a roommate or getting your first home, falling in love, having a child, planning your vacation, and even day-to-day activities like rooting for your favorite sports team are all manifestations or versions of healthy, manageable stress.

However, unhealthy stress is when you find yourself saying, "Oh, I'm so stressed." The scientific term is maladaptive stress. That is the type of stress that wreaks havoc. But the goal of life is not to live a life with zero stress. It is biologically impossible to do that. The goal of life is to lead a life with healthy, manageable stress that is productive and serves you rather than harms you.

David Ko: In your book *The Five Resets*, you emphasize the significance of managing this stress. And when you talk about toxic resilience—that's what we don't want to do. Can you talk about how you even manage that?

Aditi Nerurkar: Back in 2018, or maybe even 2019, the word resilience had a positive connotation. Now if you hear the word resilience, you bristle. You have a visceral response. Why is that? Because it's a manifestation of hustle culture, continuously striving to work harder and longer even to the point of risking your own well-being, and "resilience" became a buzzword. However, the scientific definition of true resilience is not an endurance test at all costs, it's your innate biological ability to adapt, recover, and grow in the face of life's challenges. True resilience needs a little bit of healthy stress to show itself. Without healthy stress there can be no resilience.

What our hustle culture created is *toxic resilience,* which is very different. It has morphed, and it's become something dark and sinister. True resilience honors your boundaries, understands your human limitations, and celebrates your ability to say no when needed. It really leans into the lens of self-compassion. Toxic resilience, on the other hand, is productivity at all costs.

David Ko: I like the idea of honoring your boundaries [as] true resilience. When I was younger, on a personal note, my parents used to tell me when I struggled with my own mental health journey to "power through it." It's part of the culture of many Asian immigrants. I could relate to so much of what you were saying, because even though we may have grown up on different coasts [and have] other differences, I think we had similar types of parents.

Aditi Nerurkar: There's a lot of taboo around mental health in certain communities, particularly Asian and immigrant communities. And you know, if there's one silver lining with this pandemic that we lived through, it's that a lot of these concepts are evergreen. Since we've lived through these pandemic years — individually and collectively— and we've come out of the sense of trauma it brought about, we might now be experiencing a delayed stress response. So, if there is any silver lining, it's that people like you and others in the C-suite (a company's top management positions) are understanding, recognizing, and talking about mental health. Of course, through Calm, you're a pioneer and unique because you helm an organization that focuses on mental health. But other leaders in the world are finally talking about it and thinking about it. Finally, the topic of mental health came out of the shadows and is being recognized by CEOs and business owners. Doctors have always known mental health has been an issue, but it's finally being seen and recognized, because no one is immune from these challenges.

David Ko: You're right. None of us are immune. In writing this book, that's one reason I decided to use the battery analogy—everyone from my kids to my parents could understand. We're all always checking— where is my phone's battery at? Do I have it charged enough to get me through the next chunk of my day? And so I'm using the idea of the mind as a battery and checking in with it—just like we check our phones.

Aditi Nerurkar: I love your analogy of the battery for several reasons. Along with the great resilience myth, there's a myth that we have an unlimited amount of bandwidth, brain resources used for attention. Again, it's a manifestation of toxic resilience and hustle culture. The truth is that we don't have an unlimited amount of bandwidth. We have a very finite amount which can easily get used up trying to manage your stress and burnout on a day-to-day basis. It's very easy for our inner critic to hold up a megaphone to say, "You're not doing enough, you need to do more." When you use all your bandwidth for that, it's hard to get out of your own way. So, understanding that we do truly have a limited battery life, and when we are running on fumes, like many of us are, we need to give our brain, the battery, a chance to recharge. Your body's biology is expertly designed to handle short-term acute stress. But we should be thriving and not just surviving. To do that, we need periods of respite.

Then that's another reason why this battery analogy is so poignant, especially now, because in the wake of COVID-19, we have not had a respite. We've gone through something incredibly traumatic on both individual levels and as a global whole. And the pandemic is just one disruption our generations have experienced in recent history. We have faced extreme climate disasters, humanitarian crises, and an onslaught of crises, one after the other. So how do you recharge your battery when it feels like the world is quite literally falling apart around us? I assure you, none of us are alone in wondering when and how we're going to catch a break.

It would be wonderful if we could all just go live in Bali and take a surfing vacation for six months or something, but that's not realistic for most of us. We have financial constraints, we have time constraints, we have responsibilities to our work, to our families. Some of us have to take care of elders, or sick relatives. Many of us have children depending on us. There are so many constraints on our time, that we get into a habitual routine that may be producing toxic stress. When it gets to that point, often our thought is an all-or-nothing fallacy: *Well, if I can't just check out and go somewhere, and you know, not think about my stress, why bother trying?*

Fact: It is *always* worth trying to reduce your stress. We've talked about the physical stakes you risk when your mind remains under prolonged pressure. Recharging your battery should *not* look like letting yourself get down to less than 5 percent before plugging in, but you *should* remember that any charge is better than none. You've likely been in the spot before, where you're out and about and your phone's nearly dead. If you could just charge for ten minutes, you'll have enough juice to be able to route your way to your destination. You have some goal in your head—*Let me charge until I'm at 25 percent, and then I'll be ready.* The good news is that your mental battery isn't any different. The truth is in the science; small efforts can make a big impact when it comes to managing your stress and burnout and recharging that battery. For example, a wonderful study showed taking ten-minute breaks cumulatively throughout the day helps rewire your brain and improves your state of being.[49] That's it, just ten minutes at a time—a total of maybe thirty to forty minutes a day, spread throughout the afternoon. These sorts of breaks are not just nice to have; they're essential, especially if you are someone who has one meeting after the other after the other after the other. While we can't all scale back and take it easy, you can be really intentional with your time. Schedule in three to five ten-minute breaks throughout your day to honor your break time and help recharge your battery *before* it falls dangerously low.

• • •

The innovative phrase *toxic resilience* stuck with me long after my conversation with Dr. Nerurkar. I could relate to the concept. The clarity Dr. Nerurkar speaks about what true resilience should look like struck a chord. It was a new concept for me.

I couldn't help but think back to the toxic resilience of the pandemic. We certainly saw that essential frontline workers bore the brunt of resilience in the early COVID-19 crisis, including not only those working in healthcare, but extending also to workers in education, transportation, and food services—people from all walks of life, all dealing with uncertainty, crisis, and chronic stress. After what we saw, experienced, and learned throughout the pandemic, it's imperative that we put mental health at the center of workplace policies for the health of our employees—for ourselves. But then, when we were still learning to navigate our "new normal," I knew

---

49   Jamie Friedlander Serrano, "Lie Down, Sit Still, Take a Break: Your Brain Needs a Rest," *The Washington Post*, June 29, 2024, https://www.washingtonpost.com/wellness/2024/06/29/brain-rest-zoom-breaks/.

that as a CEO, I would have to really *listen* and discern what was the best course of action in this very unusual time in business operations.

I remember sending everyone home from the office we had just rented in San Francisco. When the state of California told everyone to shelter in place, I told myself it'll only be for a few weeks. A year and a half later, the start-up I'd just founded had only met in person a handful of times, outside, six feet apart. Learning how to build community over Zoom was ... impossible. Luckily, many of us had worked together before, but we brought in people that started remotely, and it was hard to build community. Work-life balance went through the window, as we were all suddenly working full time from our homes. And for us parents, that meant working from home, where our kids were also attending school full time virtually. Many of us were getting up early to prepare lesson plans at 5:00 a.m. before logging on for a full day of work. I can't say we had a healthy workforce. It was hard.

I had our team do Zoom bingo sessions. We tried to do online activities together. But it wasn't easy.

I thought we could power through. We were wrong.

"A healthy workforce," says US Surgeon General Vivek Murthy, MD, "is the foundation for thriving organizations and healthier communities." And I fully agree, along with his continued statement: "As we recover from the worst of the pandemic, we have an opportunity and the power to make workplaces engines for mental health and well-being."[50]

It's hard, as leaders, to know the best way to approach this conversation. Which, again, is why listening is a great place to start, particularly to our surgeon general, who identified a framework for

---

50   Amy Novotney, "Why Mental Health Needs to Be a Top Priority in the Workplace," American Psychological Association, last updated April 21, 2023, accessed July 2024, https://www.apa.org/news/apa/2022/surgeon-general-workplace-well-being.

balanced workplace mental health (Figure 3.2), inclusive of five key elements that all align to bring employees a greater sense of well-being:

1. Protection from harm (including safety)
2. Connection and community (the social supports provided to employees)
3. Work-life balance (our next section)
4. Purpose and "mattering" at work
5. Opportunities for personal growth

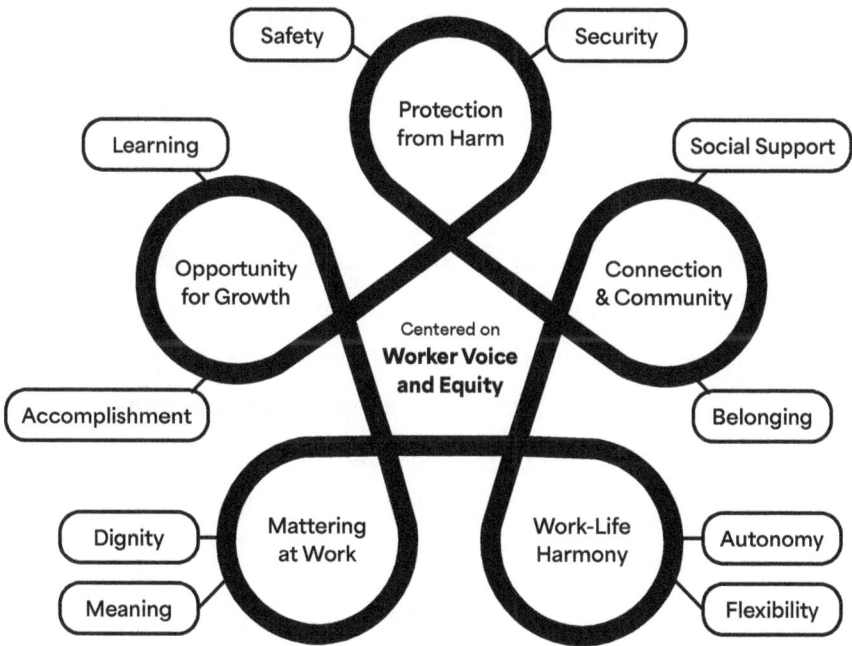

Safety / Security / Protection from Harm / Learning / Social Support / Opportunity for Growth / Connection & Community / Centered on **Worker Voice and Equity** / Accomplishment / Belonging / Dignity / Mattering at Work / Work-Life Harmony / Autonomy / Meaning / Flexibility

Figure 3.2: The surgeon general's framework for workplace mental health and well-being[51]

The global trauma of the pandemic, of what it has meant for the workplace, for us, as we are seeking balance, has a silver lining in that we are actually having these conversations.

51   Ibid.

⚡ Recharge Your Battery: Workplace Power-Ups

Even in the busiest workday, there are ways to give your mental battery a boost. Try these quick recharge techniques:

- **Walking meetings:** Suggest a "walk and talk" for your next one-on-one meeting. The change of scenery and light exercise can energize both parties.
- **Tech-free lunch:** Step away from your desk and enjoy your meal without screens. This mental break can help you return to work refreshed.
- **Desk yoga:** Try simple stretches like neck rolls, shoulder shrugs, or seated twists to release tension and increase energy.
- **Positive affirmations:** Keep a list of encouraging phrases nearby. These can be popular quotes that resonate with you, but especially when it comes to destressing while at work, it helps to keep a record of compliments that coworkers and clients have given you over time. You can then go back and read one whenever you need a quick mental boost.

• • •

Listening to Those You Lead

As a leader, I have spent years—from my time in university—thinking about what kind of leader I wanted to be. Never has it been more important to be an intentional leader.

My children, as I wrote earlier in the book, are amused by my collection of Hermès ties from my days in banking. They also love what is known in my family as the "phone book story."

The phone book story is about the time a banking director "lost it"—and I happened to be the subject of his ire at the moment. He hurled a big phone book, the old Yellow Pages—a *Manhattan* Yellow Pages. Now investment bankers on Wall Street are not usually known for their athletic prowess. He was aiming at the wall, but his lousy throw meant I actually had to dodge to ensure it missed me. When I tell this story, the first thing my kids find hilarious is there used to be these fat, heavy books filled with phone numbers where you could look stuff up—companies, addresses of friends, you name it. Pre-Google. The phone books were so thick that, if one were lobbed at your head, you'd probably get a concussion.

The other aspect of the story they're shocked by, of course, is that someone could behave that way in the workplace. The first time I told them about it, my older daughter asked, "What did you do?"

"I ducked," I said. A very Gen X response. To be honest, I was so used to eating stress for breakfast, lunch, and dinner that I shrugged and moved on. I didn't think much about it at the time. But what I did take away from the experience was that it made me think about what kind of leader I wanted to be in the workplace (for one, I knew I would never throw a phone book—admittedly a low bar). When I first moved into a leadership role, it was where preparation met opportunity. I had been reading everything I could about leadership, in addition to studying, observing, and talking to people.

Throughout my career, I've seen great leadership—and I saw styles like "the phone book guy." What I disliked about "phone book guy" the most was not that he threw phone books, but that he never listened. He didn't listen to feedback from anyone on the team. Innately, I understood that listening to my teams produced far better results. In fact, what rose to the top for me was how important it is for leaders—from frontline managers to the C-suite—to be good listeners.

When I had a conversation with John Sculley, former CEO of Apple, I realized that listening as part of leadership and the workplace was one of his superpowers.

A Conversation with John Sculley: Chief Listener

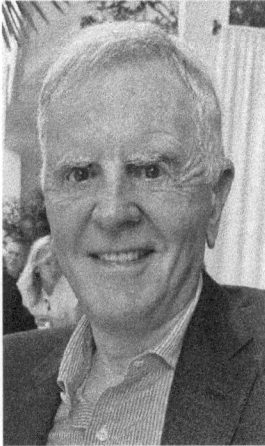

John Sculley is a businessman, entrepreneur, and investor—and innovator. He's been president of PepsiCo and CEO of Apple, and is currently involved in a number of start-ups in the tech space. He has also worked and continues to work in the healthcare industry, both internationally and in the United States. We discussed the immense stresses on both executives and employees in high-pressure business situations, as well as some of the experiences that led to how he approaches the high-stress environments where he thrives.

David Ko: As someone who has worked with so many people that you mentor in the start-up space, so many people you give advice to outside of mentorship, how do you give them advice on how to handle stress? And how do you personally handle stress in your life?

John Sculley: I think it starts with good personal habits. The reality is that, regardless of what your age is, you have to get enough sleep. You have to be healthy enough about the things that you can control. There might be some things you're born with, and there may be problems you've got to deal with. But for the most part, good nutrition, exercise, and sleep [are essential].

You will find yourself in situations which are going to overwhelm you all the time. There will always be situations where you're overwhelmed. But it shouldn't be the routine as well.

David Ko: You were at Apple, definitely a pressure cooker, and you were able to work with Steve Jobs. And he pushed you guys really hard. How did you get through some of those stressful times? And how did some of the employees get through that?

John Sculley: I would say, first of all, we believed in the dream. And that no one was better than Steve Jobs to be able to explain how he saw the world was going to be … he was gifted in his ability to describe how the world was going to change, and why Apple would be the, in his mind, change agent. Steve was the best recruiter in the world. He had this ability to recruit just extraordinary people, and he surrounded himself with extraordinary people.

So it was exciting to be involved with Steve. But he could drive everybody crazy because he was so demanding … we would have been doing something at nine o'clock, and everything was going well, and then I'd get a call [a short time later] from his assistant, and she would say he was in a different building, and she'd say, "John, get over here right away. Steve is upset." So I would head over, and he'd be screaming at people, and you know he was mad, and he wanted to fire people, and so we always took a walk, because Steve didn't like to be in an office. He liked to walk around.

So we would go for a walk and talk it out.

When Steve and I worked together, in those days people had business cards, and he said, "Let's change our business cards." So I went and thought about what I would want people to think of about me on my business card. I came up with a new title. I was still CEO, but a new title of my business card was chief listener because I think listening is a skill.

I found that you can have more impact on people and organizations, on projects, on everything if you listen carefully. You know, really listening is a development skill. I had the advantage of having the speech impediment when I was a kid up until sixteen so I had to do a lot of listening, because I couldn't do a lot of talking, and so I feel so lucky I had that advantage.

• • •

In my opinion, leadership begins with listening. Listening is, as John says, a development skill—and an underrated one at that. I believe it's foundational to a healthy work culture, one with [fewer] phone books and more listening! Some of that is partially innate for me. I don't think I've ever been a person to rush headlong into a conversation. Around the leadership table, I've always listened to our teams, leaders, and investors. Listening is about empowering your employees, building trust, gaining insights about what's happening on the ground of your organization. And in this era of an increased focus on mental health in the workplace, active listening is also a building block for empathy. It's the other side of the conversation. Just as important to engaging with someone and talking is listening to the other person. Being present and giving yourself to the conversation forces you to be in the moment, to be focused, engaged, and actively listening.

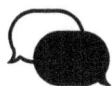

Extending the Conversation: Practice Active Listening

Though this is in our chapter on the workplace, active listening can apply to every relationship in your life. We can all be better listeners. So what are the traits of active listening?

- **Focus.** Pay attention to the speaker. Try to be present. Eliminate as many distractions as possible. Put down your phone.
- **Make sure your nonverbal clues reflect listening.** Don't cross your arms over your chest or appear "closed." Nod. Make eye contact.
- **Reflect or mirror.** "What I hear you saying is xyz ..." Repeating back or mirroring what the other person says (or what you think they said) affords the opportunity to clear up any miscommunications right away.
- **Empathize.** Try to acknowledge the feelings and perspective of the other person.
- **Do not interrupt.** Very often leaders are "bottom-line" people. Avoid the temptation to interrupt or finish the other person's sentences.
- **Ask appropriate questions.** Asking follow-up questions that demonstrate a thoughtful approach to the discussion builds trust.
- **Recap.** In the workplace especially, it's essential to finish with a recap of what was discussed and next steps.

• • •

Work-Life Balance

One Christmas the tech company where I worked gave out sleeping bags as a holiday present.

At the time, to be honest, we all found it funny. It was given to us in the spirit of a dedicated founder who spent days sleeping in the office because he was working hard on something we all believed in. It was like what John Sculley discussed in our conversation—we were building something bigger than ourselves, and everyone put in the hours. Passionate entrepreneurs and creators and certain types of people push themselves—but I promise you, even if you are founding a company, a lack of balance will eventually catch up to you. Today, I cannot imagine a company making that joke, because increasingly we recognize sleeping in the office shouldn't be our default goal. There is adaptive stress—that "good stress" we discussed earlier, and there is the "bad stress," the chronic stress that is hurting us in body and mind.

Over the last few years (and even before that), I started thinking about that question of work-life balance, of mental health, and I started to make some intentional changes as both a leader and a person. When I began working for a major healthcare organization and really focusing on the issues around healthcare and wellness—which necessarily includes mental health—and then when I moved on to Calm, the issue became more pressing to me.

I can trace the trajectory of my thinking by looking back at my annual bucket list. It's more of a goals-and-dreams list, not a list of things I want to do before I die. I've kept one since my twenties, and over the years, it has become a document that my family shares. We all leave ideas and thoughts about what it is we want to accomplish over the next year, including trips we'd take, languages we'd try to learn, hobbies we wanted to try. But in those early, high-flying years, when it was just me and my list, the bulk of my goals were about leadership, making money, and advancing my career. Now I'm pleased to say that the list is more about building a well-balanced life. It's important to put goal posts to your ambitions—it's how you actually achieve those dreams—but it's equally important to balance them with goals that are about simply enjoying the life you have and the people you're lucky to live it with.

We all know the adage that no one ever says on their deathbed, "I wish I'd spent more time at the office." I used to travel three weeks out of the month; now I try to limit travel to four or five days a month (not easy as a CEO!) and to fly home the same day if possible.

Globally, workers are placing this same emphasis on valuing their work-life balance, even above their actual salary values. In a 2021 study of nine thousand workers in the United Kingdom, 65 percent of respondents said work-life balance was more important to them than pay and benefits.[52] In the United States, 84 percent considered flexibility a key issue.[53]

However, before the pandemic, I think work-life balance was largely thought of as only a flexible work schedule (and at that, the accommodations could have been as slight as staggered start/finish times). But the pandemic shifted how we, as a global whole, look at work-life balance, especially with remote and hybrid work. In addressing this cultural shift in our mindsets around work-life balance, a BBC article reported:

---

52   Kate Morgan, "What Does Work-Life Balance Mean in a Changed Work World?," BBC.com, February 28, 2023, https://www.bbc.com/worklife/article/20230227-what-does-work-life-balance-mean-in-a-changed-work-world.

53   Shawn M. Carter and Sarah Davis, "Work Life Balance Outranks an Easy Commute and Paths to Promotion In Employee Values, New Survey Finds," Forbes.com, May 13, 2022, https://www.forbes.com/health/mind/work-life-balance-survey/.

Increasingly, employees say the idea [of work-life balance] encompasses a holistically healthy work environment that allows for an open dialogue between employees and employers. This communication enables them to address their personal lives in the context of their careers, and create the life they want ... work-life balance now is broader, deeper, and more nuanced—and it is no longer a one-size-fits-all equation.[54]

More flexibility has both positive and negative aspects. For some people during the pandemic, particularly parents facing childcare centers or school closings, flexibility may have come at a deep personal cost in terms of the stress of overseeing school lessons or cooped-up children while also pretending on Zoom—with blurred backgrounds disguising the messes in their houses—that everything is just fine. Really, once "commuting stopped, and people found themselves working in, or steps away from, their couches, kitchens and bedrooms, the veil between worklife and homelife was lifted."[55] Others found themselves caring for elderly relatives while also caring for children for the first time. Families frequently found themselves moving in together (such as young adults moving home) as adults for the first time in many years. Single people and those living alone coped with extreme isolation—especially if the workplace was a part of their social life, as it is for many of us. There were companies who expected round-the-clock logging in to try to make up for what was happening. The toll was enormous for everyone.

For others, being able to eliminate long commutes and pop in and out of a home workspace while attending to other things—and to work at night, for example, or the hours in which that employee feels most productive—was a welcome change.

---

54   Ibid.

55   Ibid.

For me, the silver lining of being in a family pod during the pandemic was the time I gained—and never would have spent otherwise—with my family. We reconnected, and I did the things that I never had time for before: having dinners at home together, instead of me taking business meetings over dinners out; spending weekends trying to keep ourselves amused; talking more; playing board games; walking the dog together more. We slowed down. I had, for the first time in my life, a better work-life balance.

However, outside the pandemic bubble, I've been finding myself wondering if work-life balance is actually achievable. The world has resumed operations, and I can feel the extra travel days creeping back into my calendar. The difference is I used to view working eighty hours a week as a badge of honor. Amelia O'Relly, whom we met earlier in the book, referred to it as "hustle culture." Dr. Aditi Nerurkar also used the term, equating it to "toxic resilience." That mindset, along with the expansion of technology and digitization, led to a blurring of work-life balance. In fact, businesswoman Betsy Jacobson is quoted as saying: "Balance is not better time management, but better boundary management. Balance means making choices and enjoying those choices."[56] One thing that has helped me bring balance to my postpandemic life is having the vocabulary to talk about where I am and what I need. I want to share with you one more excerpt from my conversation with Amelia O'Relly about the phone-battery analogy I use to talk about mental health:

David Ko: The analogy I am using is about charging our phones, and how that connects with our mind. I am curious

---

56   Abbey Slattery, "20+ Quotes on Achieving Work-Life Balance from Successful Women," InHerSight.com, last updated May 22, 2024, accessed July 2024, https://www.inhersight.com/blog/insight-commentary/work-life-balance-quotes.

to hear your thoughts around how mental health influences physical well-being.

Amelia O'Relly: I love your analogy of the phone battery because it's something so many of us can relate to, and I think you can go even further with that analogy. I think sometimes we go to charge our phones and think, "Oh my God, my battery's already dead." And it's because you are using some apps that are draining that battery, right? And so, I think if you take that same concept to personal life, I think we all have to think about whether there are things or pieces of our everyday lives that are draining our battery more. And how do we balance that? Because if you work in an environment that is constantly taking, taking, taking, it doesn't matter how much you charge yourself. You're always going to feel drained once you're in that setting, so you have to be more conscientious about how much space you give of yourself to certain things. And I think that without question, if you don't do that, I think the toll shows up physically and often mentally. We have people that burn out, and bad things happen, but we also have other people that are seemingly managing it. However, what's happening is the body is the one taking the beating, and I think it's why you see, sadly, so many executives becoming ill right when they're getting into their prime earning years, in their fifties. All these things start showing up. And I think doesn't happen overnight. It's the toll of that degree of responsibility, the expectations.

I know for me that was the case without question. And it's like compounded interest the wrong way. It's over time. What does it do? If I just take a small example, think of when an executive goes on holiday. I worked in organizations where it was frowned upon to put a sign out if you were on vacation. [It was more] "I'm on vacation. But in reality, if you need to reach me, here's my number. Here's my passcode. Here's my passport." It's like, why go on vacation? So I submit we're all responsible. Because if you can't take a few days off and truly recharge, something is wrong.

What I see happening now is that intention to at least be aware of [mental health and recharging], to talk about it, to do something about it, whereas before it was expected that you were going to do whatever it takes to succeed and to deliver.

I've been guilty of that kind of "vacation" myself. What's so interesting to me is once I started talking to people about recharging and the battery, somehow it seemed easier to understand. I am hoping, then, that helps with our next workplace issue—what happens in business when leaders don't address mental health.

The Costs of Not Having the Conversations

We are more aware now than ever before. We never used to hear of "mental health days." In certain professions (medical school residents, Wall Street, hospitality), the long hours and stress are almost the point. They're almost like professional hazing. It is also a tremendous privilege to even speak of mental health days. There are countless people, often in minimum-paying jobs with no benefits, for whom the concept of a mental health day is still not a possibility.

However, we are increasingly seeing executives embrace the fact that caring for their employees' mental health and well-being is not only just the good thing to do, but is actually also good for the bottom line. According to journal *Population Health Management*, mental health costs US companies *$200 billion a year in healthcare utilization and lost productivity.*[57]

Let's unpack that figure for a moment. When we talk about healthcare utilization, we're referring to the increased use of medical services by employees struggling with mental health issues. This includes not only direct mental health treatment, but also physical health services, as mental health often impacts physical well-being and vice versa. Remember our discussion on the mind-body connection? An employee with untreated anxiety might frequently visit their doctor for stress-related physical symptoms.

Lost productivity encompasses a range of issues, including absenteeism, where employees miss work due to mental health challenges, and presenteeism, when employees are physically present but not functioning at full capacity due to mental health issues. This could look like difficulty concentrating, slower work pace, or increased errors.

Another aspect of mental health that significantly impacts both individuals and companies is substance use disorder (SUD), which includes alcohol as well as illegal drug use. It's crucial to understand that addiction is a cost that extends far beyond the individual struggling with it. It affects families, communities, and workplaces.

Consider this: Fully 70 percent of people who use illegal drugs are employed, at least part-time.[58] But in caring for a company or a team, there is a human toll. One in ten US adults will have a substance use disorder in their lifetime.[59] The National Council on Alcoholism and Drug Dependence (NCADD) estimates that SUD

---

57   Todor Penev et al., "The Impact of a Workforce Mental Health Program on Employer Medical Plan Spend: An Application of Cost Efficiency Measurement for Mental Health Care," *Population Health Management* 26, no. 1 (February 2023): https://www.ncbi.nlm.nih.gov/pmc/articles/PMC9969895/.

58   Ibid.

59   Ibid.

costs employers "$81 billion annually through lost productivity and absenteeism, turnover and recruitment costs, workplace accidents, healthcare expenses, and disability and workers' compensation."[60] This can also translate directly to health and safety risks as hungover or preoccupied/impaired employees endanger coworkers.[61]

These aren't just numbers on a page. They represent real people—our colleagues, friends, and family members, and people like the rapper Macklemore, whom you'll hear from in a later chapter—who are struggling. And just like with other mental health issues, the impact on physical health can be profound, creating a vicious cycle that further drains our mental batteries.

It's important to note that not every issue related to alcohol or drugs is full-blown addiction. Many of us use substances to self-medicate from stress, often without realizing it. For example, while studies increasingly show no amount of alcohol is healthy,[62] many of us are using it to self-medicate from stress (and may not even be realizing we are doing so). In fact, 22 percent of people with anxiety disorders self-medicate—men more than women.[63] As Stanford Dr. Anna Lembke described it: "I'm depressed or I can't sleep, so I'm going to drink a pint or drink some wine. Or I'm anxious: I'm going to smoke because I'm overwhelmed."[64]

60 Smith, "100 Inspiring Recovery Quotes."

61 Recovery Centers of America, "How Much Does Addiction Cost Employers—and How Can Employers Help Address and Prevent Substance Abuse," June 28, 2021, https://recoverycentersofamerica.com/blogs/how-much-does-addiction-cost-employers-and-how-can-employers/.

62 World Health Organization, "No Level of Alcohol Consumption Is Safe for Our Health," January 4, 2023, https://www.who.int/europe/news/item/04-01-2023-no-level-of-alcohol-consumption-is-safe-for-our-health.

63 Drew Schwartz, "How to Tell If You're Using Substances to Numb Your Feelings," Self.com, May 15, 2023, https://www.self.com/story/self-medicating-alcohol-drugs.

64 Ibid.

This self-medication can extend beyond just alcohol and drugs to include behaviors like excessive shopping, gambling, or internet use. It all comes back to our attempts to recharge our depleted mental batteries, often in ways that can ultimately be harmful.

The costs—both financial and human—of ignoring mental health in the workplace are staggering. But there's hope. By creating an environment where these conversations can happen openly and without stigma, we can start to address these issues head-on. We can provide support and resources and create a culture where taking care of our mental health is as normal and accepted as taking care of our physical health.

Remember, our mental batteries need regular charging to function at their best. By ignoring mental health in the workplace, we're essentially trying to run high-performance machines on low power. It's not sustainable, and ultimately, it's not good for anyone— employees or employers.

In the coming pages, we'll explore more specific mental health challenges and strategies for addressing them. But for now, let's focus on the importance of starting these conversations and creating a culture where mental health is prioritized alongside physical health and productivity. After all, a fully charged team is a more creative, productive, and ultimately more successful one.

Leadership from the Top

When it comes to addressing mental health challenges in the workplace, work-life balance needs to start at the top with leadership and permeate through the whole organization. I mentioned earlier how at Calm, we start our all-hands meeting with a meditation—it's a normal part of our company culture, but I'll be honest: that first time, I was caught off guard.

Certainly, in a work capacity, I had not meditated in public. It just was not part of the corporate lifeblood and fabric of any of the places where I had worked, despite the research that supports utilizing meditation in the workplace to improve organizational culture, help employees avoid burnout, and enhance collaboration and problem-solving skills.[65] In fact, the Society for Human Resources Professionals (SHRM) has reported on how meditation and prayer rooms can improve feelings of inclusion, and how meditation programs can have concrete health benefits.[66]

Everywhere I looked around me at Calm, I was impressed with how mental health was integrated into the fabric of the company—whether that was employees gathering to listen to positive podcasts to start the day, having virtual events over Zoom, making time for meditation before meetings, or offering robust mental health benefits that complemented rich medical benefits, the company truly makes an effort to nurture employees.

I remember when one of my male employees gave me the heads-up that he was going on paternity leave. This was unheard of during my time in banking and tech. Not him notifying me, but the fact that he was taking paternity leave at all. I myself took no days off when I had my kids. I hadn't given much thought to paternity leave before then. But once I reflected, I realized that *yes*, paternity leave is just as important as maternity leave. It's *hard* to care for a newborn, for both

---

65   Joanne Sammer, "Meditation Comes to the Workplace," Society for Human Resource Management, June 11, 2014, accessed July 2024, https://www.shrm.org/topics-tools/news/benefits-compensation/meditation-comes-to-workplace.

66   Karen J. Bannan, "Meditation Offerings Can Help Employees in Difficult Times," Society for Human Resource Management, April 8, 2020, https://www.shrm.org/topics-tools/news/employee-relations/meditation-offerings-can-help-employees-difficult-times.

the birthing parent and their partner. The disparity between the paid time off granted in paternity leave in comparison to maternity leave is significant, and even more so when you begin to compare the United States's parental leave policies with that of the global workforce. The United States is one of seven countries in the entire world that does not mandate paid maternity leave.[67] The global average is twenty-nine weeks paid. And many countries offer much more.[68] Paternity leave in the United States is also offered by only 17 percent of companies. The *only* way to change mental health support in corporate America will be through leadership that says that yes, this is important. Time off after a child is born is essential. (I've since found out that despite many companies offering paternity leave these days, most men take an average of ten days or less—even if offered weeks of time off.[69])

Empathy Throughout

As diversity, equity, and inclusion (DEI) programs gain traction, employers are seeking not only a diverse workforce, including gender, race, ethnicity, age, and sexual orientation, but also people who literally think differently. "Neurodiversity" was coined only in the late 1990s by Australian sociologist Judy Singer and became a priority in the 2010s as companies faced a tight labor market.[70]

---

67   Claire Cain Miller, "The World 'Has Found a Way to Do This': The US Lags on Paid Leave," *New York Times*, October 25, 2021, last updated June 22, 2023, accessed July 2024, https://www.nytimes.com/2021/10/25/upshot/paid-leave-democrats.html.

68   IRIS Global Workforce Management, "Maternity & Paternity Leave Statistics Around the Globe," accessed July 2024, https://fmpglobal.com/resources/guides/maternity-paternity-leave-statistics-around-the-globe/.

69   Jessica Grose, "Why Dads Don't Take Parental Leave," *New York Times*, February 19, 2020, https://www.nytimes.com/2020/02/19/parenting/why-dads-dont-take-parental-leave.html.

70   Ed Thompson, "The Rise of Neurodiversity at Work," Psychology Today, May 24, 2023, https://www.psychology-today.com/us/blog/a-hidden-force/202305/the-rise-of-neurodiversity-at-work.

There is probably not a person reading this book who does not know someone who is neurodivergent. Perhaps you yourself. People may—because of media attention and more openness about it—think of neurodivergence as people on the autism spectrum. But it is so much more than that—ADHD, autism, dyslexia, and just the uniqueness of each person's brain.

In fact, in my conversation with Johnny C. Taylor, president and CEO of the Society for Human Resource Management (SHRM), we discussed that "neurodivergence" is not a simple term to define. In terms of a dictionary-style definition, it means someone's brain works in one or more ways that are different from "standard" or "normal." I don't know about you, but I have to ask myself: What is "normal"?

The challenge is to make sure that management and employees have empathy and realize that two people will never share the exact same thought process. It's our job as leaders to create empathy throughout the entire organization for one another, rather than trying to choose rigid qualifications and fit square pegs into round holes. I shared with Johnny that as a leader, I simply think that each of us use our brains in unique ways and problem-solve in unique ways (which is why collaboration and teams are so important). Whether someone is on the spectrum, has ADHD, or has another diagnosis, we can look, as leaders, for ways we can accommodate people's needs. Doing so, I believe, creates a more robust, passionate workforce. In fact, high scores in a study of "belonging" led to a 56 percent increase in job performance.[71] But I think it's also a matter, again, of having the conversations with acceptance and compassion—a first step toward a healthier, happier team.

---

71   Evan W. Carr et al., "The Value of Belonging at Work," Harvard Business Review, December 16, 2019, accessed July 2024, https://hbr.org/2019/12/the-value-of-belonging-at-work.

Policies for Positive Mental Health in the Workplace

I try to be an intentional leader. Anytime I have to make a decision for the company, I consider a variety of viewpoints in an effort to make the most intentional and beneficial decision I can. For example, when we were all so Zoom'ed out during the pandemic lockdowns, we had Zoom-free days so employees could work on their projects uninterrupted. The way I view it, meetings are an easy place to enact intentionality in the workplace. We don't have to meet face-to-face, but when we do, we should be intentional and present with each other. Not just for the sake of being physically together. The same is true of virtual meetings. When we gather as a team, it should be when the topic at hand requires that level of energy. For any other reason, you're draining your team's batteries when they could be putting that valuable charge elsewhere.

For example, even if I work on the weekend, I will be sure to set my emails to send Monday morning, because I know that even if I assure my teams that they can wait until after the weekend to respond, I am aware that an email coming from the CEO carries weight. I want employees to know they should be disconnecting from work outside of business hours, so I have to set the example.

The following are some key areas around mental well-being in the workplace and policies that can have positive impacts:

- **Flexible work arrangements:** As discussed, flexible work arrangements give employees greater autonomy to get their work done in the most efficient way for them. I should point out that flexible work arrangements do not mean exclusively working from home. It means allowing employees to take the personal time they need so they can show up to work recharged.

- **Employee assistance programs (EAPs):** These can offer substance use disorder treatment, confidential counseling, mental health resources, support networks, etc. Importantly, not only should they be available—but they should also be widely publicized throughout the company so that no one need worry about where they would find help should they need it.

- **Mental health days:** Implementing policies that allow employees to take time off specifically for mental health reasons without stigma or penalty encourages self-care and reduces burnout. Employees should be reminded that mental health days are there for a reason and to take them as needed.

- **Wellness programs:** For a long time, most wellness programs focused solely on gym memberships. More recently we've begun seeing offerings like smoking cessation programs or other initiatives focused on physical health, such as yoga classes or meditation sessions, or even providing employees subscriptions to apps like Calm. Wellness programs that provide both mental and physical support enable stress reduction in the workplace.

- **Realistic workload management:** I love that quote from businesswoman Betsy Johnson that I used earlier—time management is really boundary management. Realistic workload management is essential to the mental health of the workplace. We all understand the crunch at the end of each quarter, etc., but if a company cannot thrive while having reasonable workloads for its people, it will eventually become a toxic workplace. Boundaries around after-hours communication should be clear as well.

- **Antidiscrimination policies:** Mental health status should not be used as a discrimination tool, and promoting inclusivity and acceptance within the workplace helps reduce stigma and create a supportive environment.

- **Conversations:** This book was written to start conversations around mental health. It is my hope that this can usher in openness and communication—in families and our personal lives, but also our work lives. When managers and executives are empathic and withhold judgment, as well as encourage conversations on mental health, this reduces stigma and helps us all to be vulnerable around what's really going on with us.

Let's have a check-in on your workplace battery.

Check Your Battery: Your Workplace Battery

For this battery check, check in on how your work stress weighs on you.

- Are you setting clear boundaries?
- If you are a leader, what are you doing to ensure workloads are realistic?
- How do you feel work influences your mental battery?
- What are the clues for you that you may be getting burned out?
- What are your key stressors?
- Perhaps the most important question of all: How are you coping with workplace stress?

• • •

One of the things I have been curious about as I've written about the workplace and mental health is how other CEOs and leaders view workplace mental health and how best to help employees and teams handle stress. I was lucky enough to get to have this discussion with Jack Rowe.

A Conversation with Jack Rowe: Healthcare Innovator

John Wallis "Jack" Rowe is an academic physician who served as chairman and CEO of Aetna. Most importantly, he is my friend and mentor. A MacArthur Foundation research recipient, he is the coauthor, with Robert Kahn, of *Successful Aging*. After leaving Aetna, he became an active philanthropist, supporting aging research and other causes. I wanted to talk to Jack about his perspective on mental health from a CEO's point of view. I thought it would have changed drastically. The language has changed, but turns out, things are more similar than different.

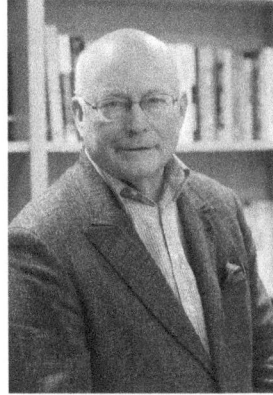

David Ko: As we talk about mental health strategies, I of course ask what do you do to recharge your mind? And how has that changed over the years?

Jack Rowe: Well, first I guess I would describe it not so much as recharging as avoiding having to recharge. Avoiding crashing.

I had a very interesting experience when I was in the research phase of my career … I'm a biophysicist. I used to do biophysics research at Harvard and at MIT. I had a laboratory that was going very, very well, and we published a peer-reviewed article in a high-quality journal once a month, twelve a year … I was working all the time, to the point where my wife took the kids and went, rented a place in Cape Cod, and invited her mother, and I would go down on weekends. But to be honest, I'd arrive on Saturday afternoon, and I'd leave on Sunday afternoon to get to the lab to check the animals.

I realized that this wasn't working for us. It wasn't working for me, wasn't working for her, wasn't working for the children. And this was not a long-term strategy that was going to be successful. So I systematically and purposefully cut back on my work. And my relationships with my family improved dramatically.

I took more time off. And the most interesting observations for me was that the quality of my research improved because I was in kind of a rut of just doing the next thing, the next thing … the next thing. This gave me time to think about what's really important here. What direction should we go in? … So I think balance is important; it's not thinking about what your recovery plan is. It's thinking about how to prevent needing recovery.

David Ko: You have had all of these leadership positions, and you have this discipline, this mental fortitude, to actually find that balance. But what about for your employees? How did you preach to them to have that balance?

Jack Rowe: There was one specific management tool that I use, that I think was helpful in this regard. I would tell them that I thought it was very, very important for them to *think* about what they were doing. And the first time they heard this, they looked at me like I was an idiot.

But I'll give you an anecdote. One day the CFO had some problem, and he came up to the floor of my office. He goes to my assistant, and he says, "Is Jack in? I need to see him. It's just going to take a few minutes. It's very important."

When she told him I could not meet with him, the CFO asked if I was on the phone, or if I was meeting with someone.

She explained, "He blocks out sessions where he just sits in the office and thinks about what he's doing and what's going on, what the company's issues are. And trust me—you don't want to interrupt him."

This anecdote went through the company ... executives have come up to me. "What's this thinking time?"

David Ko: A reminder that some of the mental health habits start from the top.

Jack Rowe: You have to decompress. In order to *think*, you have to get into neutral. Right? You have to get out of drive, and you have to get into neutral. I'm not a meditation guy like you folks at Calm. But we all understand the value of getting out of gear.

David Ko: What other advice do you have for CEOs today, as they try to handle more of their employees' well-being, especially a world coming out of COVID, but also a world with a lot of distractions and stress?

Jack Rowe: Number one is, I think, that there's never been a CEO who hasn't faced a really challenging problem in his or her company. Whether it's distress associated with COVID, the stressful nature of the job, financial stresses, whatever. But there also has never been a CEO at the end of a stressful period who felt they had communicated too much. You just cannot communicate too much.

David Ko: Do you feel that at times we should have mental health discussed in the boardroom? Or do you feel like that's something that should not be discussed in the boardroom?

Jack Rowe: I think one has to be careful about the language we use. When many people hear "mental health" or "mental illness," they think of severe, persistent problems such as schizophrenia, manic-depressive illness, or treatment-resistant depression. But what we are talking about here, and what you and your colleagues at Calm are dealing with, [are] much more anxiety and depression associated with stress. So rather than introduce the topic of mental illness in the boardroom, or the workplace in general, I think that a better strategy is to talk about stress and talk about the adverse consequences of stress. How they accrue over time, how they impair performance and one's ability to enjoy their life, and their relationships with others … it's stress.

David Ko: I like the fact that you can take away the stigma of talking about mental health by talking around stress. Now let's discuss about how physical health is intertwined with mental health. Do you feel we understand this better?

Jack Rowe: There's been more integration in large part because of the emphasis on primary care providers and a holistic approach to the patient … at Aetna I was always trying to integrate our mental health benefits with our so-called health benefits. As a clinician, I knew that a woman [who] delivers a baby [and] develops postpartum depression does not need two health plans. A man who suffers a heart attack and develops an anxiety disorder afterward doesn't need two health plans. [If] you are helping support the clinical management of these patients, you should not separate the physical and mental issues clinically or administratively.

• • •

I could talk to Jack for hours. I *have* talked to Jack for hours! I always leave the conversations fully recharged, because Jack listens with intention. He's a model CEO that reminds me that leadership comes from the top down, especially regarding mental health. Jack practices what he preaches when it comes to balance and burnout. As a CEO with a family and with many demands on my time, I feel that my conversations like the one with Jack remind me to continue to be intentional in how I care for my mental health—and that of my team.

But writing the chapter, I also thought of how Zoom'ed out we have all been, how drained by the turbulent times we are living in. As a tech guy, I realize that gets me thinking about how we can use tech to help us with our mental health.

Chapter Four

Technology and Mental Health

―――――

For Better and Worse

> The human spirit must prevail over technology.
>
> **—Albert Einstein**

The intersection of tech and mental health, for me, starts at my fingertips. Literally.

I wear devices that measure elements of my health—most importantly, sleep. As someone in tech, I love data (and cool toys). And the devices I wear enable me to analyze whether I am getting quality sleep, and that further lets me analyze the lifestyle choices I make. What am I doing to ensure I have true, restorative sleep?

When I looked at the data, it became clear that alcohol completely messed with my sleep. Even if I got enough hours of sleep, after a night of cocktails, I still felt tired the next day. The data showed I wasn't reaching REM sleep. Alas, I'm not twenty-five anymore, and I can't drink like I did when I wore Hermès ties. My data made it easier to make changes and get a better night's sleep.

Today, everything from watches to rings to fitness and mental health apps can provide real-time data that measure how we're doing. Whether it's slowing our heartbeat with a biofeedback program or my ring letting me know I actually did not get the REM sleep I needed, technology is making it easier for us to monitor our health.

I see unprecedented potential in what technology can tell us about our health and in what ways it can support us in our mental health journeys. I think technology can help us make healthcare more accessible and easier, and give us more control over our data and health decisions—all at our fingertips.

But I also cannot help seeing the dangers and pitfalls of technology—the seas of notifications awaiting our kids. The curated "perfection" that we scroll through and the effect it has on all of us. Technology is the ultimate double-edged sword because of both the outsize benefits and dangers.

It also isn't going anywhere. Technology is ubiquitous and here to stay. The genie is definitely out of the bottle. For me, as a leader in an industry that is squarely at the intersection of healthcare and tech, I always try to figure out how I can help. Ever since joining Calm, and especially since my conversation with Jack Rowe when I was at Zynga, I've been hyperfocused on finding ways to use technology to improve our mental health and do good in the world. However, what I've realized while working on these solutions is that I can't fix something no one is willing to even talk about. How can I get people to start talking about their mental health—both in the workplace and otherwise—without it being thought of as weird? Ironically, one of the first conversations I had with my parents about mental health that had a huge impact on me was silent.

The Dining Room Table

Sometimes we listen without words.

When I was young, I used to travel to South Korea to visit family, including my grandmother. I appreciate that not only is she still here with us today at one hundred years old, but also that I've had those opportunities to get to know her and to spend time in the culture of my parents and grandparents. To be honest, I felt like I straddled two worlds a bit. In the United States, where I grew up, I was one of a handful of Asians in my hometown. I didn't always feel as if I fit in. Meanwhile, when I visited Korea, it was easy to tell I was American—maybe the way I dressed, or nuances in how I spoke Korean. I didn't quite fit in there either.

Now, as an adult, I've mostly figured out my place in the world. I don't worry about fitting in. When I visit Korea and my family there, it is now with a different eye, on the lookout for ways I can help my grandmother, to make her life as easy and happy as possible. My mother, as is common in the culture of Korea, is her caregiver—and I see what a challenge that can be. I try to pay attention there, too, because caregivers have their own stresses.

On one of my visits, I was struck by my grandmother's dining room table. When I walked in and "listened" to what that table was telling me, it was a tale of the difficulties of aging and the stresses of keeping track of health.

My grandmother's table had become a sea of paper and Post-it notes. They were reminders—what time to take what medication, notes of things to remember to tell the doctor, blood pressure readings in an elderly scrawl. The table was no longer the center of the home, a place to eat with loved ones and talk. It had transformed into a care center, a place that caused stress and great concern.

The sight of the table and the problem it represented rolled around in my head for a while—there had to be a better way. Technology could help; I was certain of it. Why couldn't an app make our healthcare portable and trackable?

I'm not the only person in technology thinking about how we can use tech as a force of good. I had the privilege of speaking with Carl Nassib, who pivoted from the NFL to a new career—one where he is using technology to help. What follows is some of our conversation.

A Conversation with Carl Nassib: On Self-Acceptance and Purpose

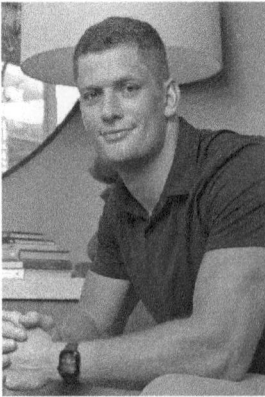

I enjoyed my conversation with veteran NFL defensive end Carl Nassib. While playing in the league, he announced his sexual orientation on Instagram and, for the first time, publicly opened up about being gay. As the first active NFL player to come out, Nassib's decision marked a significant milestone in professional sports. His openness not only garnered support from the league and teammates but also provided crucial representation, particularly for LGBTQ+ youth in sports. In 2023, he retired and went on to share a vision and purpose by creating the app Rayze, which connects volunteers (especially the tech-savvy younger generation) with opportunities, discovering in the process a new purpose. He's definitely a rebel. But an innovator too.

David Ko: Can you talk a little bit about the process of self-acceptance? And can you elaborate on the journey that you had first, as you talked about in your Instagram post, coming out to your close family and friends?

Carl Nassib: There were three processes. The first one was just self-acceptance. [The] second one was coming out to my family, and then third was coming out to the world.

I knew that I was not straight at a very young age, like thirteen or fourteen. But I grew up Catholic and dealt with so much Catholic guilt. I tried to be straight but couldn't hack it. So when I was twenty-three, I essentially had a conversation with myself, and after years of praying and trying to be straight, I was like, "You know what, Carl? You gave yourself ten years of this … thinking of God wanting you to be straight. If that was possible, you'd be straight right now." I finally took the burden off of myself. I stopped really hating myself. And I just like, you know, this isn't a choice, and I didn't tell anybody for a couple of years. It just took a little bit of a while to figure it out, and then I came out to my family a couple of years after that, which was amazing.

So the first two processes of coming out, really, were first acknowledging myself, then coming out to my family. The third part was a little more strategic. I put a lot of thought into it. I knew I wanted to do it publicly. I didn't want to have somebody else control the narrative. I wanted to live an out, free life, but I didn't want to be outed. I didn't want to go on a date with somebody I was in a relationship with and be worried about someone seeing me, and then I couldn't control it. So I knew that I wanted to break the news publicly.

But first, I knew I wanted to be in a position where I was financially stable, that no matter what happened, that I would be good to go for the rest of my life. I signed a $25 million deal with the Raiders.

And $17 million of that was guaranteed. And then, after I got that, I said, "Great! Now I can do it."

I came out in my house in Pennsylvania. I knew that I wanted to be secure there. With my friends and family close by, 'cause I just didn't know what was going to happen. And everything was absolutely beautiful. I couldn't really have asked for anything more. And my teammates, my coaches, the NFL, the media, fans. I mean, they were fantastic. I think they really appreciated the way that I came out. I think they appreciated the fact that I came out with a massive donation to a very important nonprofit [he made a $100,000 donation to the Trevor Project]. I think they appreciated that. I didn't come out with a brand deal to monetize off my sexuality. I really didn't want anybody to get the notion that I was doing this for personal gain. I wanted to do it for the next generation of people coming out, that they might not have as hard a time as people in my generation and a generation before me. And I think I succeeded. I think it was really well received, and my teammates said that they loved the way that I did it.

David Ko: How did you prioritize your own mental health during that period? I mean, from friends and acquaintances I know from the world of sports, that was not a conversation for a long time.

Carl Nassib: I don't remember hearing anything about mental health, even in college. I really started first hearing that when I got to the NFL. I know I had heard about PTSD for veterans. That was something that I would hear stories of, and that really made me sad, but I didn't hear too much about anxiety and depression, as like a medical diagnosis. I learned a lot more about that after getting in the NFL. I think I didn't know the science of it.

Luckily, you know my family ... we all just talked till the cows come home ... I've been very blessed in that way. We're happy people.

And I do not think my family had a history of some of those issues. I learned more about others' mental health journeys.

But I think so much credit goes to athletes, because especially football players are seen as such strong ,masculine people, and that you always want no cracks on the ship. So for somebody in that position to break down those barriers, and I don't know who did it first … I think it was a collective thing, but for athletes, especially in the NFL to be trailblazers, and accepting those conversations, I think, was really big.

David Ko: One of the topics we are covering in this book is the concept of purpose. You've made a pivot after the NFL. I would love if you would share about that.

Carl Nassib: I think that I'm very lucky, having something to transition to. Something that I'm very, very passionate about, which is not super common. I am extremely goal-oriented and motivated, and that is a very common thread for athletes. So when a lot of athletes do make the transition to a post-professional-athlete life, they might not have something like my company Rayze. In the NFL, we were told, "You are your business," and that's how I feel about being an entrepreneur. I have to drive the ship. I am my business still. So I feel very lucky that I can make this transition. And what excites me about Rayze is we're solving problems.

• • •

In my life, I have sometimes found even slightly personal conversations and revelations difficult. Carl's courage in a world where there are still people who are not fully accepting of the LGBTQ community just filled me with awe, on top of how he's leveraging tech in such a positive way. But the other amazing thing about Carl was that innovative career pivot.

He found out younger than I did that finding your purpose makes such a difference in your life and the lives of others.

Technology and Mental Health: Can It Help Us?

I wanted to take a moment to talk about technology, engagement, and access.

When I cofounded Ripple Health Group, it was because I saw that caring for ourselves and others can be fraught with challenges. In fact, it was Jack, again, who shared with me his belief that the problem in healthcare is a combination of trust and engagement. Many people do not trust the system, and coupled with a lack of engagement, they do not adhere to healthy regimens and habits. Many of the things that could really bring about wellness—activities that doctors and experts urge us to consider and then actually *do*—are about making real changes, whether that be exercising consistently, eating a healthy diet, giving up bad habits, making time for restful sleep, and so on.

The problem is that most people—including myself—have very short attention spans. We do things in the beginning but don't keep it up. It's like the classic January 1 gym membership. We start out on those treadmills, ear pods in, running to our favorite playlists, on January 2. We do it again on the third. But by the end of January (if we even make it that far), fitness has been squeezed out of our lives by our busy schedules, by the January winter doldrums, by whatever it is that keeps us from fully engaging and committing to our health.

Jack's theory was that if we got folks to engage more deeply in their healthcare via technology and apps the right way, then we could actually make more people healthier. That could create less of a burden on our dysfunctional healthcare system. We could get people to the right care they need to be healthy.

Gamification and Our Health

Over the years, we have watched as gamification has invaded every aspect of our lives. With the tech that exists just in my phone, I can get rewarded for nearly everything—learning a language, making purchases on certain platforms, logging what I eat into certain apps, etc. Fitness apps encourage us to compete against ourselves and others; there are apps for children to earn points by learning responsibility caring for virtual pets. Whether you're putting your points toward acquiring free products, or future discounts, or simply a higher ranking in an app, the gamification of these digital trackers is proven to enhance user engagement, making usage of the app a habit in and of itself. With gamification, game-design elements are used in nongame contexts by leveraging motivational techniques and engaging users in activities that promote desired behaviors, such as the following:

- **Rewards and achievements:** Probably the most well-known tactic, gamification can include points, badges, and rewards for completing health-related tasks, such as exercising, eating healthily, or attending medical check-ups. These rewards can motivate individuals to stick with their health routines.

- **Progress tracking:** Visual progress bars and milestones help users see their improvements over time, making it more likely they will continue with their healthy habits.

- **Behavior change:** Gamified systems can help in forming new habits by providing consistent feedback and rewards for repeating healthy behaviors, such as daily step goals or drinking water—or even getting outside.

- **Stress reduction and mental health:** Games and apps that incorporate mindfulness exercises, relaxation techniques, and stress-relief activities can help users manage mental health more effectively.
- **Mood tracking and journaling:** Gamified elements in mood tracking apps encourage regular updates and can provide insights into emotional well-being, helping users to recognize patterns and triggers.

Of course, as we've discussed, the internet and tech can have a major, negative impact on a person's well-being. But the inverse is true too; when we use tech to gamify healthier habits, then we're making tech work for our lives, and not the other way around. Fitbit—the wearable, watchlike fitness tracker—is a great example of how gamification improves one's engagement in their well-being and leads to healthy habits. Humor essayist David Sedaris said this about his Fitbit: "This year, I got a Fitbit. You walk 10,000 steps and it sends you an email saying, 'That's great! A lot of people don't walk that far. Do you think you can walk 5,000 more steps?' And so I say, 'I bet I can!' A week ago, I walked 60,000 steps. That's 25.5 miles. I'm completely obsessed. It's like a sickness; I've been Fitbit-ten."[72] (But like I wrote earlier, don't be afraid to start with a short walk after dinner!)

The opportunities at the intersection of technology and health-care are just beginning. I believe we can make a difference in how people care for their minds—the batteries that power everything else. It starts with getting the tools into everyone's—and I mean everyone's—hands.

---

72   David Sedaris, "Stepping Out," *The New Yorker*, June 23, 2014, https://www.newyorker.com/magazine/2014/06/30/stepping-out-3.

Technology and the Access Conundrum

One of the things technology does is make a service that was hard to come by easier to access. By offering scale, matching, customization, security, and streamlining in nanoseconds, we can access the world and what it has to offer like never before. Think about arranging a taxi ride before there was Uber or ordering a book online before there was Amazon. It was harder, took longer, and depending on where you lived, was potentially even impossible. As devices get cheaper and data more affordable, technology has been a great equalizer. But—as of yet, at least—not when it comes to mental health support.

I know the data regarding access to mental health in this country, and the statistics are dire. My mission is to leverage all the ways technology can help get mental health support to everyone in the world, not just the people who can pay. The primary barriers to making this a reality include

- imbalanced access to support and services;
- a shortage of mental healthcare providers and geographical/distance barriers;
- financial constraints;
- cultural stigmas and communication differences;
- systemic barriers, including insurance/healthcare systems;
- lack of awareness.

Indeed, one of the primary concerns is the scarcity of mental healthcare providers, especially in rural and underserved areas. Throughout my career, I have always lived near large cities. A privilege of that (and of my excellent insurance) is that should I need a healthcare provider—including for mental health—while I might be put on a waiting list, there will not be an issue of being unable to locate a professional within a reasonable drive from my home. For that matter, the fact that I have a car and can drive myself and my family to our healthcare appointments is a privilege as well. If, for some reason, the provider I need is outside my network, I even have the means to pay for that out of pocket.

We talked about Uber earlier. People tend to think of locating a therapist as a bit like calling for an Uber driver. If I just press a button or type a search into my insurance plan's website or Google, one will magically show up. People who think that way have likely never looked for a psychiatrist, or there's a level of privilege they enjoy that's afforded them a different, less common reality. In fact, more than half of the counties outside of metropolitan areas in the United States do not have a practicing psychiatrist.[73] In addition, "160 million Americans live in areas with mental health professional shortages, with over 8,000 more professionals needed to ensure an adequate supply."[74]

Even if you live in an area with a supposedly adequate number of providers, waiting lists are long. According to the National Council of Mental Wellbeing, average wait times are about six weeks, but for specialists or areas with access issues, that can stretch to months.[75] Access is a major issue in mental health.

In my conversation with psychiatrist Ken Duckworth, chief medical officer for the National Alliance on Mental Illness (NAMI), he agreed access is a significant problem. As he challenged:

> You try finding a child psychiatrist who accepts insurance within a hundred miles of you. And that's not the child psychiatrist's fault. We take wonderful human beings. We

---

73   Nathaniel Counts, "Understanding the US Behavioral Health Workforce Shortage," The Common-wealth Fund, May 18, 2023, https://www.commonwealthfund.org/publications/explainer/2023/may/understanding-us-behavioral-health-workforce-shortage.

74   Counts, "Understanding the US Behavioral Health Workforce Shortage."

75   Nina Chamlou, "What to Do on a Therapy Waitlist," Psychology.org, August 2, 2022, https://www.psychology.org/what-to-do-on-a-therapy-waitlist/.

send them to medical school. We give them a quarter of a million dollars of debt when they're in their early thirties and starting a family. And then, we say, would you like to take an underpayment from a health insurance company? Or would you prefer to make a lot of money and just get paid privately and have nobody check your paperwork?

We haven't made it very easy for people to participate in an insurance system that fundamentally undervalues mental health.

We take for granted if we have a heart problem, we will be able to access a cardiologist relatively quickly. Yet somehow, when it comes to mental health, we see a very broken system.

We saw these access issues during the COVID-19 pandemic. On the one hand, telehealth meant people could do therapy online; however, there were still shortages of providers. During the pandemic, 84 percent of psychologists who treat anxiety disorders saw an increase in demand,[76] as well as increased waitlists. Research also indicates that while, for example, young people find teletherapy comfortable because they are digital natives, not all people do, including older adults and certain other segments of the population.[77]

People covered by Medicaid—and, to a lesser extent, Medicare—also struggle to find providers that accept their insurance, in large part because of low reimbursement rates. One study found that in Oregon, more than half of the mental health providers listed in network directories of Medicaid-managed care plans did not actually take Medicaid

---

76 American Psychological Association, "Demand for Mental Health Treatment Continues to Increase, Say Psychologists," October 19, 2021, https://www.apa.org/news/press/releases/2021/10/mental-health-treatment-demand.

77 Mental Health America, "Teletherapy During COVID-19: What the Research Says," accessed July 2024, https://www.mhanational.org/teletherapy-during-covid-19-what-research-says.

enrollees.[78] This has profound implications for equitable access, as Medicaid is the nation's largest payor of behavioral health services.

Overall, financial barriers pose a considerable obstacle to accessing mental healthcare. Many individuals lack adequate insurance coverage for mental health services, or they may face high out-of-pocket costs for therapy sessions, medications, or hospitalizations. This financial burden—on top of the stigma that we've been discussing—often forces individuals to forgo or delay seeking treatment, worsening their mental health conditions over time. I also had a conversation with rapper Macklemore for this book—you'll get to read more of his story in a moment—but during our discussion, he shared that when he went to rehab for substance abuse the first time, his father managed to pull funds together for the full cost of treatment. They were not a wealthy family, and that was a huge sacrifice. That kind of cost is crippling for many.

But let's say that finances aren't much of a barrier for you. As I said, I have the privilege of being able to pay out of pocket if necessary for any medical care I or my family might need, but just like everybody else, I'm still going to face a wait time to be seen. This is a type of systemic barrier, and for people who do also face a financial barrier, it compounds to make it even less likely they'll seek treatment. Systemic barriers can also include complicated referral processes, lack of coordination between primary care and mental health services, and inadequate integration of mental healthcare into overall healthcare delivery.

Our latest venture at Calm, a product called Calm Health, takes aim at systemic barriers within the healthcare system. Calm Health enables organizations to offer to their people customized experiences for each individual, based on where they are in their mental and physical health journey. So for example, when a new person opens

---

78   Counts, "Understanding the US Behavioral Health Workforce Shortage."

the app, they are asked—in a warm and engaging way—to fill out a personal, confidential screening —the same one professionals use to diagnose depression and anxiety—about their health conditions, what mental health concerns they may have (such as anxiety, loss of a sense of joy, etc.), as well as physical health concerns like high blood pressure, chronic illnesses, and more. In addition, the user will be asked about their mental health every three or four weeks—the better to track changes over time. The convenience of apps and technology is but one *tool* in our mental healthcare toolbox, but in terms of access, an app can be with you twenty-four seven.

Other access issues can be cultural and linguistic barriers. People want to talk to others who make them feel comfortable, who have a foundational understanding of their identities. Often, that means trying to find a therapist who looks like them, understands their cultural norms and the way they grew up, or who understands the unique pressures of their gender identity. Yet according to the latest demographics survey by the American Psychological Association, 84 percent of all US therapists are white.[79] About 40 percent of the US population is not white.[80] This disparity in representation can create additional challenges for accessing mental healthcare, particularly for minority and immigrant populations. Language barriers may hinder effective communication between patients and providers, leading to misunderstandings or inadequate treatment. Cultural differences in beliefs about mental health can also influence whether individuals feel comfortable seeking professional support, further limiting access to care.

All these factors reduce anyone's ability to engage fully in their medical and mental well-being, and compounded over time, these

---

79   American Psychological Association, "Psychology's Workforce Is Becoming More Diverse," 51, no. 8 (November 1, 2020): 19. https://www.apa.org/monitor/2020/11/datapoint-diverse.

80   Ibid.

systemic and cultural barriers that form through generations devolve into a lack of awareness and education about mental health issues and available resources. Not everyone knows when sadness seeps into depression. When do you need professional help?

This is where technology shines. By using the power of data and technology, people can be empowered to monitor and recharge their batteries. Tools like Calm Health are a first line of defense. More than just making you feel better because it helps you check in on yourself and monitor how you are doing. Calm Health will also let you know if you may need to get professional help. In fact, if someone is seriously in mental health trouble and reports thinking of self-harm, the app will direct them to a suicide hotline (and it's always good for us to pause here for the reminder that if you or someone you know is thinking of self-harm, that is a crisis and needs immediate help—you can find a list of resources in the appendix). The app can also refer you to a therapist to talk to. Or perhaps it will provide digital support to supplement a community, such as Macklemore has within the twelve-step program.

I am immensely proud of the passion for mental health our team has devoted itself to, to create our products—and being in the technology space, I know that there is real promise in using technology to care for our mental health.

When Technology Can Drain Us

When Facebook launched, most of us thought it would be a place to share pictures of our kids with our family far and wide. This was before the proliferation of social media, which is now ubiquitous. US adults spend an average of four or five hours a day or more on our phones.[81] Teens and tweens report similar numbers.

In the book *The Anxious Generation: How the Great Rewiring of Childhood Is Causing an Epidemic of Mental Illness,* author and psychologist Jonathan Haidt discusses how toxic social media is (separate from simply being on the internet). According to the Centers for Disease Control and Prevention, 20 percent of kids twelve to seventeen years old have had at least one major depressive episode.[82]

I see it with my own kids. I don't want a sea of notifications on my phone (a sea that is often a tsunami, frankly). I turn them off for most apps. But when my teens wake up, the first things they see on their phones are hundreds of notifications from the apps they use most. Teens all over the world will rise and wonder what they missed overnight. Who liked what post? What did that person say in the comments?

In my conversation with Randima Fernando from Center for Humane Technology, he said:

> We are very much conditioned by our environment and the people around us, like our friends, coworkers, and family. But then you've got the smartphone, which masquerades as one of your closest friends. It's always with you. And it shapes your thinking and your behavior. This invisible relationship has profound effects and makes it much harder for us to be mindful. It changes you. It changes us collectively. It changes all our interactions. And it changes culture along with our values.

---

81 Stacey Vanek Smith and Darian Woods, "How Much Phone Time Is Too Much Phone Time? Scientists Research Digital Addiction," NPR.com, August 13, 2021, https://www.npr.org/2021/08/13/1027317245/how-much-phone-time-is-too-much-phone-time-scientists-research-digital-addiction.

82 Maura Kelly, "How to Calm the Anxious Generation," Harvard Public Health, March 20, 2024, https://harvard-publichealth.org/mental-health/jonathan-haidt-on-countering-negative-effects-of-social-media/.

I always tell my kids to aspire being comfortable enough with yourself that you do not need social validation of who you are and your choices. When we do not do that, technology veers toward toxicity.

While I was talking with Dr. Aditi Nerurkar, the stress and burnout expert, she discussed our collective habit of doomscrolling:

It's just a natural inclination … again, it's not you. It's your biology. It's the way for you to keep feeling safe when we scroll. What are we doing? We are feeling a sense of stress, and it's our night watchman. Back evolutionarily, when the tribe slept there was a night watchman who would scan for danger. And now we are all our own night watchman. We're feeling a heightened sense of stress. We're hypervigilant, and it's our primal urge to scroll. We are trying to feel safe and feel a sense of self-preservation. And so we start scrolling. That's what you know. Doom scrolling is powered by the same machinery that powers our stress response.

If this digital anxiety is primal in its own right, then what do we do about it? Dr. Nerurkar advises keeping your phone ten feet away from your workstation, for example, so it's out of reach, and thus, checking your phone becomes more *intentional*. We all know about falling down a digital rabbit hole, and we emerge three hours later because the algorithms were on steroids.

Recharge Your Battery: Try a Digital Detox

Every year, people around the world participate in a "Screen-Free Week."[83] They take a digital detox, as more and more research shows we are stressed by the barrage of texts, social media, emails, news, etc. Many of us, career-wise, can't do a screen-free week, unless it's our

---

83   ScreenFreeWeek.org: https://www.screenfree.org/.

yearly vacation. But we can detox on the weekends, or even in the evenings. For example, I do not leave my phone on at night, and do not check it in the middle of the night, even if I wake up.

A few benefits of a digital detox include the following:

- **Reduced FOMO.** For many of us, we've gotten so used to being on top of the news, work, social media, etc., in an instantaneous way that we have the fear of missing out. If we are not refreshing our social media feeds or our news browser every few minutes, we might be missing something. A digital detox can slow this down and offer a respite or cure for FOMO.[84]

- **Better sleep.** Most of us know the blue lights from our cell phones are not conducive to restful slumber.[85] This is why it's wise, even if you think you cannot do a digital detox for a day or week, to certainly do a digital detox for the hour or two before bed.

- **Increased productivity.** There has been much discussion about how the constant bombardment of notifications and the resulting interruptions have shortened our attention spans (and those of our kids). A digital detox can give you back uninterrupted time for better focus and productivity.[86]

- **Improved mental health.** Relentless scrolling can increase anxiety and depression. A digital detox gives mental health a break from the impacts of blue light, doomscrolling, and the like.[87]

---

84   Cleveland Clinic, "How to Do a Digital Detox for Less Stress, More Focus," November 23, 2021 https://health. clevelandclinic.org/digital-detox.

85   Rob Newsom and Abhinav Singh, "Blue Light: What It Is and How It Affects Sleep," SleepFoundation.org, last updated January 12, 2024, https://www.sleepfoundation.org/bedroom-environment/blue-light.

86   Cleveland Clinic, "How to Do a Digital Detox for Less Stress, More Focus."

87   Ibid.

Continuing with our metaphor of recharging our mental health battery, Dr. Nerurkar added:

> We want to be more intentional at night, too. How can we refill our battery creating a digital boundary at bedtime? That means keeping your phone off your nightstand. Study upon study has shown us that [many] people in the United States and likely globally check their phone first thing in the morning. They're looking at headlines. They're looking at social media. And all of that has an impact on your dopamine, on all of the brain cascade and your stress response because your brain doesn't recognize the difference between a calamity 3,000 miles away and something happening close to you. Your amygdala starts firing ... so creating digital boundaries is more important now than ever. This is not about being a digital monk, but when you think about how can you recharge your battery, it's about reconsidering your relationship with your digital device. We have boundaries and every other relationship in our lives with our spouses, our colleagues, our children, our family members. Why don't we have a boundary when it comes to the relationship we have with our phone?

As a parent, I am well aware, as my daughters are now teens, that you pick your battles. One of the battles I've tried to fight the good fight on is no phones in the bedroom at night. Put them away. Create that boundary.

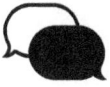

Ask Yourself (or Your Kids):

- Why are you reaching for your phone?
- Why are you scrolling right now?
- How long have you been on your phone?
- Do you need this information, or is this a reactive habit? Are you scrolling to procrastinate?
- If you're scrolling out of habit, what can you do instead right now?
- Do you feel better about yourself after being on that app?

Check Your Battery

Let's see how your mental battery relates to technology and your phone. Let's conduct a little social experiment. Put your phone in a drawer in another room—turn it off. While you're at it, collect the phones of your partner, kids, etc., and put them in the drawer too.

Now go about your activities—your normal household activities—for an hour. Keep track of each time you feel anxious that you can't check your phone. How often did you stop? Did you panic a little? How about your kids?

Now check that mental health battery. Do you feel better for your hour away from your device? Were the first few minutes hard on you? But after fifteen minutes or so, did you feel a shift?

Did not being able to check your phone for an hour reveal to you it's an obsession?

Consider your *relationship* with your devices and tech—and ask yourself: Are they helping or hurting your mental battery?

Chapter Five

Our Biggest Mental Health Challenges

Recharging from the Tough Stuff

> Promise me you'll always remember: You're braver than you believe, and stronger than you seem, and smarter than you think.
> —*Christopher Robin, Winnie-the-Pooh*

We, not they.

Dr. Ken Duckworth, of the National Alliance on Mental Illness, really brought something powerful home to me when he said during our conversation, "COVID made mental health a 'we' thing, not a 'they' thing."

We saw it all around us.

Dr. Duckworth said, "People saw their kids getting depressed, going to Zoom school but not really paying attention. People felt cut off, economic distress, grief. All of a sudden, we had a conversation where you couldn't miss it."

Yes. The conversation was everywhere. From the media to Zoom calls, to whispered discussions with our partners at bedtime. In this chapter, I want to first remind readers that we're trying to recharge; we're trying to honor our mental health and care for it the way we care for our phones, conscious of that battery. We cannot cover the many serious ways in which our mental health can suffer and conditions that may need intervention—topics best covered by doctors. I urge anyone to avail themselves of resources, hotlines, twelve-step groups, and more to get the help they need—don't forget to review the appendix for a list to get you started.

Here, though, in this chapter, I wanted to examine some of the big mental health challenges of our times, common to many of us. To the *we.*

It's all around us.

Let's talk about it.

Stress and Burnout

Some of us thrive on stress.

I know a woman who pushes tasks off intentionally so she can be a whirlwind and get it all done under the stress of a ridiculous deadline. I'm not too sure of that approach. But I *do* know there are different kinds of stress—and not all stress is bad.

There is the stress that wreaks havoc with our bodies. Upset stomachs, headaches, all the things we discussed in the mind-body chapter. But there is also *eustress*.[88] It is the "good stress." Think of a

---

88   The American Institute of Stress, "What Is Stress?," accessed July 2024, https://www.stress.org/the-good-stress-how-eustress-helps-you-grow.

marathon you've trained for and you are the starting line, or a new job you are excited to start—you feel a little anxious, elated, stressed, but it's a motivating kind of stress that pushes you forward. Eustress keeps us motivated and working toward goals.

I'm a big believer in this kind of stress. I was giving a speech at NYU, where I talked about how I hoped the graduates had the grit to find their way and the courage to find their "why." There will be stress in figuring out both—it's undeniable, and it's a good thing. Stress builds resilience, creativity, tenacity, and greatness. NVIDIA CEO Jensen Huang also spoke to a group of graduates at Stanford, and in his speech wished the students "ample doses of pain and suffering."[89] Not something you usually hear. His point was, "Greatness is not intelligence. Greatness comes from character. And character isn't formed out of smart people, it's formed out of people who suffered."

It's when stress becomes chronic that it becomes unhealthy and can have an impact on your mental and physical health. It is the real drain on our mental health battery—like having way too many apps open all at once for a long time.

People with chronic stress often include caregivers, the over-worked, those with long-term health conditions, first responders, those struggling long term with unhealthy relationships or family issues, those struggling financially, and many others. Far too many of us live in a state of perpetual stress. It is not the stress that builds greatness, grit, or a diamond. It's the stress that's harming us.

After the pandemic, the American Psychological Association conducted a research study on stress in America in 2023 and found the following:

---

89   Podium VC, "Nvidia CEO Jensen Huang on Building Resilience with Pain and Suffering," YouTube (1:39), April 2, 2024, https://www.youtube.com/watch?v=vOvQSqY7Jgc.

- Around three in five adults (61 percent) said people around them just expect them to get over their stress.
- Nearly half (47 percent) said they wish they had someone to help them manage their stress.
- Some adults (36 percent) said they don't know where to start when it comes to managing their stress, and a third (33 percent) said they feel completely stressed out, no matter what they do to manage their stress.
- Two-thirds of adults (66 percent) said that, in the last twelve months, they could have used more emotional support than they received, and around a quarter (26 percent) cited the need for a lot more support.
- More than two in five adults (44 percent) said they don't feel anyone understands what they are going through, and more than half (52 percent) said they wish they had someone to turn to for advice or support.

And as "another consequence of a society under stress," they reported that nearly "three in 10 adults (28 percent) said they have struggled with or had difficulty planning for their future in the past month because of stress," and that "a third of adults (33 percent) said they have too much stress in their day-to-day lives to think about the future."[90]

Burnout is that next level of stress. It is a state of emotional, physical, and mental exhaustion caused by prolonged and excessive stress. We usually think of it in terms of very stressful jobs, but there are other reasons people burn out. Common denominators can include a lack of control, a sense of hopelessness, exhaustion, and more.

---

90   American Psychological Association, "Stress in America 2023," accessed July 2024, https://www.apa.org/news/press/releases/stress/2023/collective-trauma-recovery.

I return to my conversation with Dr. Aditi Nerurkar. She is, after all, a stress and burnout expert. She shared with me the idea of the resilience myth. She said, "Resilience is protective, but it's not enough to prevent burnout."

I think that's important to hear. Because just as I, as a kid, did not know how to prevent panic attacks, many of us learn this myth of resilience, that "power through" mentality I had for years on Wall Street. *I just need to be tougher, more resilient, have more grit.* But the fact is, resilience alone will no longer be enough when your battery is barely holding a charge.

To return to the idea that respect for mental health in the workplace has to start with leadership, Dr. Nerurkar offers this piece of advice: "As you are engaging with your employees, overcommunicating about mental health, stress and burnout is really the way forward, because you really can never overcommunicate, because everyone is struggling. Assume that when you're engaging with someone, that it is the rule rather than the exception, because of the data."

Once again, the "we"—if we are to recharge as individuals, as families, as companies, and as a society, these are the conversations that will help us. Dr. Nerurkar added the salient point that helping those around us—our loved ones, coworkers, employees, neighbors, and friends—assumes you've already created a culture of psychological safety. There should be no taboo or stigma around sharing stress and burnout concerns. When she made these statements, I realized this whole book is my attempt to communicate the importance of all these concepts.

Research again and again[91] demonstrates that *just talking* about our problems helps. And it does not have to be to a therapist. Talking

---

91   Eric Ravenscraft, "Why Talking About Our Problems Helps So Much (and How to Do It)," *The New York Times*, April 3, 2020, https://www.nytimes.com/2020/04/03/smarter-living/talking-out-problems.html.

to friends, and even at times venting on the internet (the hashtag #TalkingAboutIt was started as a way for people to discuss mental health), can improve one's ability to recharge.[92]

I'll confess: when I get stressed out, I talk things out with myself. When I was younger, the voices were overwhelming and caused more anxiety. The playback kept me up at night. I kept replaying conversations that happened during the day; it didn't end. As I got older, I realized that when I start constantly talking to myself, I'm stressed. Once I recognized this, I started to use my internal monologue to help me work through my stress. Now, instead of the overwhelming noise in my head, I harness the energy to talk through issues with myself. Trying to see all points of view, talking out all the scenarios. The voices no longer cause me stress; they help me work out what's stressing me out. Conversations help recharge our battery, even when they are solo.

Depression: More than Sad

Just like some stress can be good, sadness is a healthy emotion. In one of my favorite Disney movies, *Inside Out*, sadness is a signal for help. Extraordinary growth, empathy, and appreciation comes from sadness. It's OK to feel sad. Depression is different. It feels constant. You feel hopeless and worthless.

According to the World Health Organization, 280 *million people* worldwide have depression.[93] It's still misunderstood in that too often, well-meaning people around those who are depressed will urge them to just be happy, to just look on the bright side. In fact, this is one way in which burnout and depression differ. In some ways, they can

---

92   Ibid.

93   World Health Organization, "Depressive Disorder (Depression)," March 31, 2023, https://www.who.int/ news-room/fact-sheets/detail/depression.

look very similar. Exhaustion, lack of interest in things that ordinarily would make someone happy, headaches, sleep issues, etc., can be part of both. However, burnout usually pertains to a circumstance—a job where a person is putting in eighty hours a week for an unpleasant boss, caregiving a parent with dementia, etc. But depression, while it can be related to circumstances, can be more pervasive and without a specific catalyst.

There are numerous tools and questionnaires online that ask questions such as, "Over the past two weeks, how often have you felt little interest or pleasure in doing things you usually enjoy?" as well as questions about how well you are eating or sleeping, in addition to gauging your energy levels. When depression is severe, it can lead to an inability to perform the activities of daily living and thoughts of hopelessness and self-harm.

Recharging from depression requires a multipronged approach that may include medication, talk therapy, or even hospitalization. However, starting the conversation is the first step—remember the "we," not the "they." You do not need to be alone.

Anxiety

Every single one of us is anxious about something. It could be a presentation, finances or household worries, insecurities about work or a relationship, or any number of things, from the small ("I am stuck at this light; will I be late to my appointment?") to the large ("Am I going to be laid off?").

Anxiety is a natural response to stress, characterized by feelings of worry, nervousness, or fear about an imminent event or something with an uncertain outcome. While occasional anxiety is a part of life, persistent and excessive anxiety can interfere with daily activities and might indicate an anxiety disorder. Understanding anxiety and learning effective coping skills are crucial for managing its impact on mental and physical health.

Anxiety could include generalized anxiety disorder (GAD), panic disorder (raising my hand here), social anxiety disorder, and specific phobias (everything from heights to clowns to spiders). The symptoms of anxiety can be both psychological and physical. Psychological symptoms include constant worry, irritability, restlessness, and difficulty concentrating. Physical symptoms can range from rapid heartbeat, sweating, and trembling, to headaches, dizziness, and digestive issues—all those symptoms we discussed in the mind-body chapter. These symptoms can be debilitating, significantly impacting someone's quality of life.

In terms of recharging, when you suffer from anxiety, you want a go-to technique that can help those feelings to subside. I know someone who suffers from panic attacks, and besides a prescription medication for very bad episodes, she has learned to plunge her face in a sink of ice water—a method that works for many.[94] A friend's nephew, who has Asperger's, loves his weighted blanket—even as he is now a six-foot-three man. Someone else's recharge station might be using the Calm Breath Bubble or reciting a specific song or mantra. I encourage you to try some of the suggestions throughout the book if you struggle with feelings of anxiety to find what works well for you. And remember—it's not about being perfect, but being consistent. You've got this.

---

94   Bonnie Zucker, "4 Ways to Cope With a Panic Attack," Psychology Today, September 25, 2023, https://www.psychologytoday.com/us/blog/liberate-yourself/202309/4-ways-to-cope-with-a-panic-attack.

The Good, the Bad, and the Ugly of Coping

When we're stressed, we cope. Or at least, we try to. There are good ways of coping, and you already know there are some pretty bad ways too. Good coping for me looks like taking the dog for a walk, taking a break, and my *one* small indulgence in having ice cream some nights. Bad coping skills were my years of smoking cigarettes, eating late-night Chinese food, and having a scotch to fall asleep.

When we think of the big mental health challenges we face, we can recharge in a good way—or in a not-so-good way. We're going to hear from rapper Macklemore at the end of this chapter, and he will discuss his issues with, and recovery process from, substance abuse disorder. That is a common coping mechanism. Now he surrounds himself with his own and a chosen family/support group that supports his recovery—and he meditated just before our conversation.

Consider your coping skills. Some that work against us include the following:

- Substance use or abuse
- Denial (pretending the problem will go away is never helpful)
- Overeating or undereating
- Self-harm
- Isolating and withdrawing from friends and support
- Workaholism
- And more

One of the problems with unhealthy coping skills is they can actually make problems worse. If someone isolates from their support network, then their feelings of isolation and loneliness will only worsen. If someone uses alcohol as their only stress reliever, eventually they will require more and more alcohol to get the same relaxation effect—not to mention that alcohol disrupts sleep, is dehydrating, and can actually increase anxiety or depression. I often wonder if, had I been able to talk to a peer or a trusted teacher about my panic attacks, that would have taken away some of their "power." Perhaps I would have discovered it was not so unusual—and I was not alone.

Ways to recharge that can improve your mental health include these:

- Exercise (and it can be as simple as a thirty-minute walk three or four times a week)
- Mindfulness
- Meditation (yes, even if you don't like sitting still)
- Good sleep
- Healthy eating (yes, I will advocate for eating a pint of ice cream to nurse a broken heart—but not every night for a month)
- Connections—friends, family, group therapy, support or twelve-step groups, places of worship, etc.
- Pursuing hobbies and other positive outlets for stress
- Therapy
- Talking with trusted friends
- Journaling
- Positive self-talk
- Visualizations
- Getting out in nature
- Breathwork
- Yoga
- Prayer
- Practicing gratitude

⚡ Check Your Battery

- This battery check is about giving your stress level a score. From the list below, choose which stress statement and corresponding score you identify with most:
- 1 = Not very stressed at all; "I'm chill"
- 5 = Feeling stress and anxiety throughout the day, losing some sleep, not feeling myself
- 10 = I feel like my brain is going to explode, and I can't relax

• • •

Now consider your go-to coping skills. What are your healthy ones? What about the not-so-healthy? Try adding one new healthy coping skill to your routine this week. Just one thing! (And maybe try cutting at least one not-so-good one!)

A Conversation with Ben Haggerty, a.k.a. Macklemore: The Rapper in Recovery

Ben Haggerty, stage name **Macklemore,** is an American rapper, singer, songwriter, activist, and creator of the golf and lifestyle apparel brand Bogey Boys. He is also a founder of the Residency, which seeks to support emerging hip-hop artists from low-income backgrounds, offering them workshops and mentorships, as well as other support.

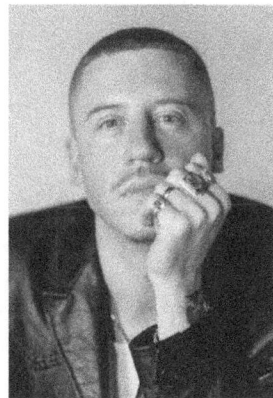

At the 2014 Grammys, Macklemore and his producer Ryan Lewis won Best New Artist, Best Rap Album (*The Heist*), and Best Rap Song and Best Rap Performance ("Thrift Shop"). He's gone on to create many hits since then. But in our conversation, what struck me was how humble he was and how open about his addiction and recovery.

David Ko: I love how you use your platform to talk about in the same way we do about what's so important: society, mental health, addiction. I truly appreciate the vulnerability of that conversation.

Ben Haggerty: You know it. I like setting the intention of just what do I have to offer, and all I can offer is my truth, my experience, my strength, and my hope, and then, wherever that goes from here is out of my control. But anytime I sit down and talk about addiction, or just my story in general—spirituality, meditation, mindfulness—I just hope to be a conduit to something greater than myself. So that's my intention.

David Ko: I love that … you know you talked about some of those early experiences when you were fourteen, with some of your first experiences with alcohol, and I was hoping you could shed a little bit more light on that day, or maybe just events leading up to it. Your early story and then your journey in recovery.

Ben Haggerty: At fourteen years old, where I think people were starting to experiment a little bit with drugs and alcohol, I went to my parents' liquor cabinet and took a shot of vodka, and then I took two, and then I wondered what four would feel like, and pretty soon I had taken twelve shots and hopped on the bus downtown, stumbling. Almost got in a fight, went to McDonald's, and threw up in the trash can, ran from the cops, and that was the beginning of my not-very-successful career drinking alcohol and doing drugs.

David Ko: Can you talk about some of those pivotal conversations that influenced your decision to go to treatment? Because it's just such a big step. Was it hard accepting that help?

Ben Haggerty: I was at a rock bottom—and I've had numerous rock bottoms since, and you know, hopefully I don't have any more. But at the time, I was addicted to opiates, and it wasn't even a long run with opiates. That's how addictive they are. I had been on a plethora of different things. And my life had always been unmanageable when using drugs. But once I started with the opiates, I really lost a next level of control where I think also that any sort of connection, any sort of spirituality, any God, any higher power spirit, whatever you want to call it, had completely vanished. I had no serotonin. I had no happiness. The only thing I had to live for was to get high, which … it wasn't even getting high anymore. It was maintenance. All of a sudden, the party kind of ends, and you're chasing that feeling that you first had when you first tried it. That's gone. And at that point, I was just trying to not be dope sick.

And I remember one day being in the studio and going outside, and it was a beautiful Seattle summer day, and I was just sobbing. You know, everything about this day was perfect. These are the days that we live for in Seattle—July, and finally sunny, and I thought, "Oh, my God … I'm living right by Green Lake at the time, and everything should be okay, and nothing was." I was so, so, so broken.

Shortly after that, I was with my parents, and I'm trying to hide it. I don't know why I was with them. I usually vanish from everybody, but for some reason I was around them. And then maybe I put together a couple of days clean, or, you know, got off the opiates and switched to something else. My dad took me out to the porch and asked me the very simple question of: "Are you happy?" It wasn't like, "You need help." It wasn't "What are you doing with your life?" It was just, "Are you happy?"

David Ko: That resonates as I've been writing this book to have these conversations ... "Are you happy?" Because I think in today's day and age, so many of us aren't. It's just such a simple question, but such a powerful one in so many ways.

Ben Haggerty: Yeah. And I think even the idea, you know, as I've gotten older, I've considered the concept [of] happiness, right? Because happiness is fleeting. But I think that we almost have this obsession with happy, which ... at the time, it was the question I needed to be asked, but to go deeper into it, the real question is, *Are you fulfilled?*

Fulfillment is a lasting process. Happiness just comes in and out. There's moments of happiness, there's moments of sadness, and that's all part of the human experience. But do you have a through line of fulfillment? Is there something that is keeping you rooted to your purpose? It's keeping you rooted to your principles, your morals, your ethics, who you are as a person, your integrity, and that's what I had lost, and happiness is a by-product of being rooted in those things.

David Ko: How have you thought about your own mental health? In your own journey?

Ben Haggerty: When I think of mental health, it's such a broad term right now. I like to kind of narrow it down. I guess I think that my problems exist in my head.

Now, when I get on my little meditation cushion behind me, and I sit and get quiet, I consider, What is the root of my misery? What is the root of my obsession or control, or wanting things to be different? It all starts up here in my head, and when you can track those thoughts and quiet them down ... then you have a toolset that helps deal with the mental health, and I think that for the disease of addiction it starts in a place of self. It's rooted in self-centeredness. That's where the disease thrives. So the more that I can get outside of myself, and what I think that I want in this moment ... you know, *if this person would just act this way, if my kid wouldn't have done that, if that offer would have gone through.* If, if, me, me, wanting things to be different versus the true place where mental health flourishes, [which] is in acceptance.

But how do we get to acceptance? It's a process, and again, it's fleeting. It's why I love the game of golf, and it helps my mental health because I see damn, really, the game is never going to work out like you think it should. I finally hit a good shot, and the ball is going to trickle off the green, and I'm going to get stuck in the bunker, and get a triple bogey. And in my head I'm like "that should have been a green in regulation." I should have had a birdie putt, and now I have a triple, and my round's over. But you have to deal with where the ball lies. That's why I love the game, and you know, our shots in life aren't always going to end up on the green. They're going to be like, oh, that should have been that, that should have been this, etc... and that's where our insanity flourishes. That's when, all of a sudden, we're out of pocket. We're out of spirit, and we're not able to be true vessels to something that connects us to where we're supposed to be in this moment.

David Ko: You pointed out something that is also core to this book's purpose. When I think about the mind, I tried to use a battery analogy. What are some of the things that you do to recharge? With your schedule, everything you have going on. What are some of the things that you do to recharge?

Ben Haggerty: I have been lately getting outside more and more. Not even golfing. Just going outside. I've been taking my shoes off. I've been trying to ground, get centered with the earth, feel the vibration through my body, actually get quiet in nature, and that's something that I've never really done, and that's been super important for me, just in terms of getting oxygen to the brain.

I have a studio in the basement. It's easy for me to get my kids out the door and then to come down here and sit in front of a computer making a beat or writing raps, and it's still a process. And as beautiful as creativity is for me, and it is important for mental health, it can become a goal, right? It's like finishing the song. What's this going to be? Or who's going [to] like it? These thoughts start popping in the head. And that's actually what disconnects you from the real, pure creative process, which is just making art for the sake of art. But if I don't have the balance of going outside, if I don't have the balance of, for me, being of service to others, I don't get outside my head.

• • •

I know I will think about the questions *Are you happy?* and *Are you fulfilled?* long after this book is done and published.

Ben's openness and vulnerability about his struggles with substance use disorder was humbling. He also had shared about his support group, about his openness with his children, about his sobriety and its importance. I consider myself mentally strong, but would I have the courage to be as vulnerable with my daughters as he is with his children and those around him? I'm not sure. I can relate to his golf-game analogy as someone who loves golf (he's a better golfer than I am, I can tell you). In life, we have to play the ball where it lies, not where it "should" be. Acceptance is a powerful tool in our mental health toolbox.

Chapter Six

The Difficult Conversations

You Good?

> Daring greatly means the courage to be vulnerable.
>
> **—Brené Brown**

I have, at different times, asked my father questions about his own life—not the life I know about, but the life before he became a father. Our parents all have these "other lives" we may not know much about. About their mental health—what they found difficult, how they survived or overcame the obstacles in their path. For children of immigrants, it can often be complicated.

I cannot say that my questions resulted in answers. Sometimes the "hard" conversations we want to have don't have the results we want (which doesn't mean we should not try again). However, it has been my experience—and one of the reasons I wrote this book—that very often, we don't even know how to begin the conversation, what to say, how to ask. If we are the one with a problem or needing help, for example, we might not know where to begin.

Why are the conversations about our mental health so difficult?

The Fear Factor

When I had my conversation with Johnny Taylor, he mentioned that, at least in corporate America, we still face difficulties when it comes to understanding mental health. As he said to me, "If you have something that is contagious, stay home." However, he then went on to point out that if someone told their supervisor they needed two weeks off because of depression, there is not a visible feverish flushed face, no flu test with a red line indicating the employee is sick. We can't "see" it or quantify its severity. Yet as we discussed in a previous chapter, during the pandemic, we "saw" it around us. Mental health was a real problem we needed to address. However, the nature of mental health and its personal perspective often make us afraid to even raise the conversation. We fear offending others (something we will discuss in the next section). We fear not having the right words. We fear we are unequipped to say the right things.

Fear runs both ways, of course. More than half of people with mental illness do not receive help because of stigma or discrimination.[95] They would rather suffer in silence than admit they have a problem. However, the silver lining to the COVID-19 pandemic may have been that it pushed discussions into the forefront. In Great Britain, 32 percent of workers are comfortable talking about workplace mental health with their supervisors postpandemic compared to 14 percent

---

95   American Psychiatric Association, "Stigma, Prejudice and Discrimination Against People with Mental Illness," accessed July 2024, https://www.psychiatry.org/patients-families/stigma-and-discrimination.

before.[96] In the United States, that number postpandemic went up to over 50 percent.[97]

The more holistic, healthy, and open response to mental health issues today is a far cry from when families kept such things secret. Randall Park's mom did not talk about her isolation as a new immigrant unable to speak the language of her new country. My parents never talked about their struggles. But even as mental health is talked about more in the media, in our children's classrooms, and in the workplace, there still exists a prevalent stigma around having these conversations, as we've talked about in this book. Societal norms sometimes mean there is deep fear of admitting mental health issues—which are seen as weaknesses. Some of our fears are associated with family or cultural dynamics. Or we may see siblings or friends just once or twice a year, and we do not want to "ruin" the mood with heavy conversations. We put the conversations off—or worse, we never have them.

For example, I know many people in my age group who are now facing issues with their parents needing extra help—or perhaps showing signs of forgetfulness that could be a safety issue. Yet we may avoid the hard conversations with them because we simply don't want to upset our parents or grandparents.

Combined with these lingering fears of judgment or discrimination, there is also fear of being vulnerable, especially in the workplace or in families or cultures or settings where being resilient, tough, or stoic is emphasized. Consider how normalized it was for years to teach our sons it wasn't OK to cry, or the responses that seem almost copied-and-pasted from person to person when you go through a

---

96   Megan Carnegie, "Is Workplace Stigma around Mental Health Struggles
      Changing?," BBC.com, August 23, 2022, https://www.bbc.com/worklife/
      article/20220819-is-workplace-stigma-around-mental-health-struggles-changing.

97   Ibid.

more public period of stress, such as a divorce or death in the family: "It gets better" or "They would want you to just be happy."

We've all been on both sides of this equation: not wanting to speak up, for fear of others' reactions, and avoiding the conversation for fear of saying the "wrong" thing.

We Don't Have the Words

Sensitivity Issues

This fear of not saying the right thing is a common sensitivity issue. Again, we have all been in the position where someone we know has experienced a profound loss, a personal tragedy or setback, or any type of situation where, for many of us, knowing the "right" thing to say is difficult. So we may avoid the situation.

This may not even be about an acquaintance or person at work who has experienced something negative; it could be in our own families. I'll raise my hand and say I don't always know how to broach topics about boys or school pressure and friends with my daughters. And so, sometimes, I don't bring it up.

We Don't Know Our Feelings

Another reason we may avoid the conversation is that we may not have the words in terms of our own feelings. For a variety of reasons, including family dynamics and upbringing, sometimes we may not have these conversations because we ourselves do not know what our emotions are. For people raised to be stoic, for example, they may not even realize when they are sad because they have been taught not to recognize or acknowledge those feelings. This can be especially common in people who have experienced trauma.

The following figure is Dr. Robert Plutchik's Wheel of Emotion,[98] designed to help people who may not be able to find the right words for their emotions to recognize what it is they are actually feeling. If you are a parent, you might remember a time when you were really, really angry with your child—maybe they stayed out an hour past curfew. But alongside the anger might be fear—you just may not articulate that.

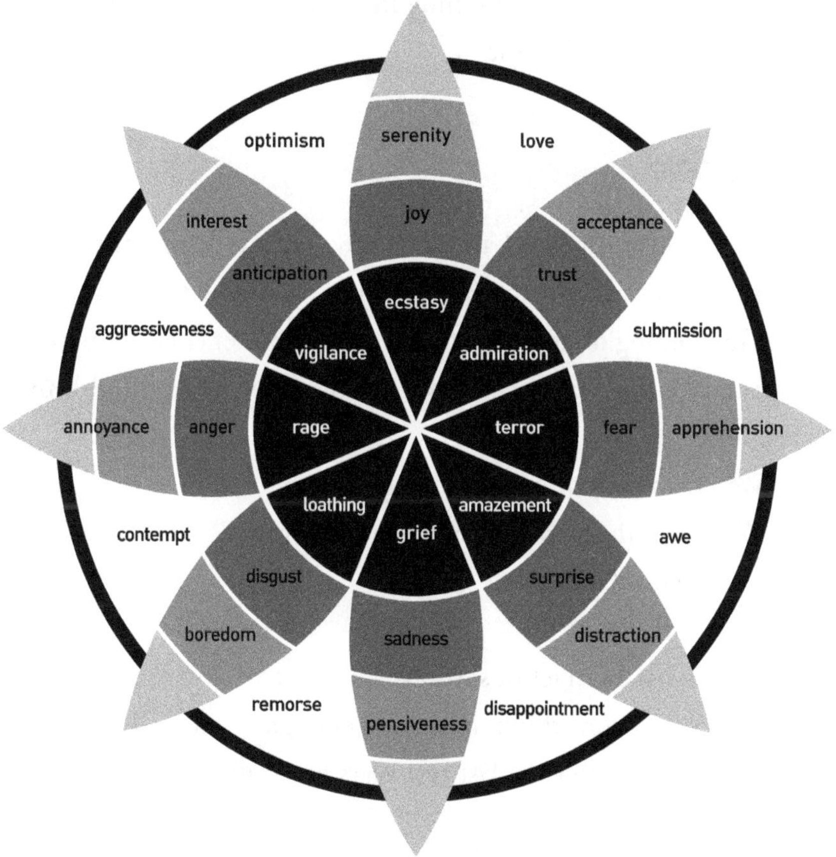

Figure 6.1: The Emotions Wheel is a visual tool that maps the spectrum of human emotions, showing how they relate to and stem from one another. By exploring this wheel, you can develop a deeper understanding of your feelings, leading to greater self-awareness and insights into your thoughts and behaviors.

---

98   Hokuma Karimova, "The Emotion Wheel: What It Is and How to Use It [+PDF]," PositivePsychology.com, December 24, 2017, accessed July 2024, https://positivepsychology.com/emotion-wheel/.

There are other versions of the emotions wheel out there, but they all boil down to the same issue. Many of us have shoved our feelings in a box or were never taught to even recognize what are feelings are. We may find our feelings overwhelming at times. Regardless, sometimes we avoid the difficult conversations because we cannot articulate what it is that is bothering us, how we are *feeling*. The more work we do to really examine what we are feeling in the moment, the easier it will be to communicate about it.

You Good?

I'm not a hugger. In fact, I am not always great at letting the people who matter to me, like my friends, know just how important they are. (I'm working on it.) Therefore, I am the poster child for why we sometimes do not have the conversations about mental health that we should.

We say to each other, "You good?"

We expect the answer to be, "Yeah, I'm good."

And then we move on.

You good?

It's a social contract of sorts. We all agree to smile and nod and go on our way. I don't think that's good enough anymore. I have been guilty of it—and after the last few years especially, I know I can do better.

What is the implicit contract of "Are you good?" It's that you will give me a superficial answer, and we can both move on with our day. Except this book has been filled with some fairly meaningful conversations and sobering statistics. Here are a few more:

- 6.8 million Americans suffer from generalized anxiety disorder.[99]
- 6 million Americans suffer from panic disorder.[100]
- 7.1 percent of the population has social anxiety disorder.[101]
- 9.1 percent of us have a phobia.[102]
- 16.5 percent of Americans have a substance use issue.[103]

We are the walking wounded and are afraid to admit it.

So we don't ask the question, and we don't volunteer that everything is not good. We each are consumed with our own "stuff" we're dealing with and may not feel we have the bandwidth to take on someone else's "stuff."

You good?

Yeah, I'm good. You?

Yeah, same.

We're not talking about it. So, then, are any of us healing? And what can we do about it?

Some of the most powerful experiences of this book have been the conversations I have had. Sometimes I already knew the person I was speaking with; sometimes I only knew them from the book they wrote or the media they did. However, what was true in each case is they gave me their time, and when I asked them questions, I gave them space to answer.

---

99   Anxiety and Depression Association of America, "Anxiety Disorders—Facts & Statistics," accessed July 2024, https://adaa.org/understanding-anxiety/facts-statistics.

100   Ibid.

101   Ibid.

102   Ibid.

103   Substance Abuse and Mental Health Services Administration, "SAMHSA Announces National Survey on Drug Use and Health (NSDUH) Results Detailing Mental Illness and Substance Use Levels in 2021," January 4, 2023, https://www.samhsa.gov/newsroom/press-announcements/20230104/samhsa-announces-nsduh-results-detailing-mental-illness-substance-use-levels-2021.

What if we offered that space to the person we asked, "How are you?" What if their answer was "good"—and we followed up with "Great, how's your battery level? Or "What percentage is your battery right now?" Now we may get a different answer. Now we have an obligation. We might have to engage. We might have to problem-solve. We might simply have to offer compassion. But the conversation now requires something of us.

Johnny Taylor of SHRM shared a story about a friend in high school who died by suicide—something that often triggers "what ifs" from those left behind. Johnny shared that if his child said she was fine, and he suspected she was not—he would dig deeper, and not have a superficial conversation, because that friend's death deeply affected him. Digging deeper beyond "You good?" is an active conversation—it asks that we engage more fully.

I still haven't had that deeper conversation with my father. While it's not a mental health conversation I crave, per se, it's the desire to engage fully with the man I admire most in the world. To hear directly from him about the moments that mattered most. What was the most stressful decision he had to make? What was it like to move to the United States? Did he ever find himself short of breath in the shower? Like Johnny, I want to dig, but like most of us, I'm slightly afraid to do so.

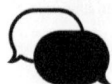

The Conversation

I thought it might be good to share some questions and statements we can all use to help start difficult conversations. I know I use them. One thing to remember is to approach any conversation with empathy and compassion, and offer space and listen without judgment.

- You say you are fine, but I want to be sure you are being honest with me. Are you really OK?
- What can I do to support you right now?
- Is there anything worrying you right now?
- How are you sleeping?
- What's been on your mind recently?
- How are you coping with your day-to-day workload?
- How is your work-life balance?
- Do you feel rested when you wake up?
- What are your main sources of stress right now? Is there something I can do to help you?
- How do you usually cope with stress?
- Are there activities or hobbies that help you relax?
- Have you ever talked to a mental health professional about what you're going through?
- Would you consider seeking professional help if needed?
- Do you feel that you have access to the mental health resources you need?
- What are you doing to recharge your mental battery?
- Are there any routines or practices that help you feel recharged?
- Have you been taking time for yourself and your own needs?
- How has your physical health been?
- Do you have any goals or plans that excite you?
- What are you looking forward to?
- How do you feel about the future?
- What level is your mental battery?

It can be equally scary to admit you might need some support or help. Here are some ways to start this conversation.

- I'm having a tough time with _____ right now.
- I am struggling with anxiety; _____ would help me.
- I've been feeling really overwhelmed lately, and I think it might be affecting my mental health.
- I've noticed some changes in my mood, and I wanted to talk about it.
- I haven't been sleeping well, and it's starting to worry me / make me feel not like myself.
- I've been feeling really anxious, and it's hard to manage.
- I've been struggling with feeling down.
- I've been having a tough time coping with stress.
- Lately, I've been feeling uninterested in things I usually enjoy.
- I've been having some negative thoughts, and it's been hard to shake them.
- I'm finding it hard to concentrate. I notice myself making mistakes.
- I feel like my emotions are all over the place.
- I've been really stressed out. What do you do to manage stress?
- How do you stay positive when you're feeling down? I could use some tips.
- I think I need someone to talk to about my mental health.
- My battery is at _____ now.

• • •

A Conversation with Harold S. Koplewicz: The Youth Advocate

When it comes to tough conversations, you couldn't ask for a better navigator than **Harold S. Koplewicz**. Dr. Koplewicz is the founding president and medical director of the Child Mind Institute, and one of the nation's leading child and adolescent psychiatrists. He is known as an innovator in the field, a strong advocate for child mental health and a master clinician. His mission is to help the millions of children—as many as one in five—struggling with mental health or learning disorders. As a parent, I wanted to talk to him about some of the harder conversations and challenges of parenting our children today.

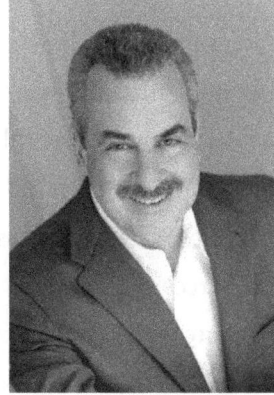

David Ko: Talk to me about the work you are doing right now—particularly in the area of mental health treatment and prevention.

Harold S. Koplewicz: I lead the Child Mind Institute, a national nonprofit dedicated to transforming the lives of children and families struggling with mental health and learning disorders. We do this through care, education, and science, where we're developing tomorrow's breakthrough treatments. Key to this is our pursuit of biomarkers—which are characteristics of the body that you can measure—so that we will be able to distinguish one child with a psychiatric illness from another. It's important to remember, psychiatry is the only discipline of medicine that doesn't have an objective test. There is no x-ray, no blood test. There is no EKG or strep test. And I, along with many other people, [am] looking at MRIs and CAT scans and EEGs and physical fitness and genetics trying to find the Holy Grail, so to speak, because if we have an objective test, parents will feel much more confident in the diagnosis. Treatment will get more precise. Stigma will disappear.

Our researchers are sharing their data globally and leading the open science initiative. I'm only hoping that we can accelerate the pace of discovery so that I'll be around for that in my lifetime.

Much of the Child Mind Institute's work today is preventative. We have developed a series of free, evidence-based video and print resources called *Healthy Minds, Thriving Kids* that caregivers and educators can use to teach their kids critical mental health and coping skills. We think of this as mental health fitness. We are teaching kids foundational mental health skills: understanding your thoughts, understanding your feelings, managing emotional stress, mindfulness, and relaxation skills.

I can remember a time when I was a kid where the only thing they had us do in the gym was square dancing! And then in fourth grade, President Kennedy said kids have to be physically fit, and we started doing jumping jacks and push-ups and sit-ups.

Physical fitness mattered. But the fact that American children don't need to know what mental health fitness is just doesn't make sense to me … every year, kids should review these five skills and teachers should … teach them, because that's what builds resilience and makes kids more robust. Mental health is health. We are so grateful to the state of California for helping us bring this initiative to students.

David Ko: Talk to me a bit about mental health issues we see in kids today.

Harold S. Koplewicz: We know that, in the U.S. alone, over 17.1 million young people will have a mental health disorder by age 18. But right now, only about one third of those millions of kids get treated. For those who do seek help, the average time between the onset of symptoms and any treatment at all is over eight years. Early intervention can change the trajectory of a child's life. We all want more kids to get the care they need, and one major barrier to seeking help is stigma. I think this is a moment when people are finally able to talk about these disorders, and I'm hoping that the more we talk about it, that health insurance is going to change to cover mental health care so that there will be real parity. God forbid you get cancer. We should cover that, and we do. And if you get depression, which is much more likely, your insurance should also cover it.

The American Academy of Pediatrics has finally said that the most common illnesses of childhood and adolescence are mental health disorders, not infectious diseases. That means we have to expand our army. Pediatricians have to become part of the first line of defense and routinely learn how to make the diagnosis of depression, anxiety, ADHD, and autism.

David Ko: As someone in tech, as someone who specifically is trying to find ways technology can help our mental health, I know you have some thoughts about that as far as kids and mental health.

Harold S. Koplewicz: We're very fortunate. We have a very smart and, I think, assertive US surgeon general, who has tackled things like loneliness and certainly making us question social media.

If we look at the fact that kids and young adults between ages ten and twenty-four who died by suicide was about five thousand, which is probably more than those who died from cancer and asthma and heart disease all wrapped up in one. But then the suicide rate jumped to six thousand by 2018, which means an already incredibly high mortality rate went up, and the number of kids who showed up in emergency rooms for suicidal thoughts or suicidal behavior went from 600,000 in 2014 to 1.2 million in 2018—which means, instead of every minute, every thirty seconds kids are feeling that way.[104] So we should look at what was happening in society that might be the cause of that increase. You know, we didn't change the water supply, and we didn't change the telephone wires. I think the only thing that really changed was that we started holding these devices in our hands that connected us to every human on the planet 24/7. While the Internet is absolutely a phenomenal resource in so many ways, it's a bit of a jungle. And so the way you should think about it is that there are wonderful fruits and vegetables in that jungle, but there are also poisonous snakes.

And right now, parents are the only people who regulate it—and they must be good about enforcing limits with their kids. We also started to notice how much more kids were using the Internet during COVID-19. We found out in our studies that kids who used it for more than six to eight hours a day, if they had a mental health disorder, they were more symptomatic.

Most specifically, if they had depression or ADHD, their symptoms got worse. So is that toxic? It was a toxic agent in the same way that marijuana is a toxic agent for people who have anxiety, they are more likely to get panic attacks, etc. So, I certainly think that social media, I think also cable news, can leave our children exposed 24/7.

[I think of the divisiveness in our country now …] I think kids must be protected from that. For example, I tell parents all the time—don't fight in front of the kids. You really want to have it out? Go into your bedroom, close the door, and whisper. Don't make anxious kids more anxious. So that's definitely part of it. I think also, we're making some progress. I think we're identifying kids earlier. And that's good because treatment works.

---

104 CDC, "Suicide Prevention," accessed July 2024, https://www.cdc.gov/suicide/facts/data.html.

David Ko: The part about social media and cable news resonates. How do you recommend we have those conversations with our children about that?

Harold S. Koplewicz: Certainly we want to model good behavior. After COVID, it was very hard for people to put their phones down. But dinner typically in America takes a very short amount of time. So, in those twenty or twenty-five minutes, if you're going to sit with your kids for dinner, you are all going to take your devices and put them in a basket somewhere on the counter away from the table. No one, even if you're a surgeon—someone can cover you for twenty-five minutes—no one's going to die if you put your phone away.

And you're going to practice having conversations. And how do you do that? I think most kids could use some advice on that. First of all, I think it's up to us to teach our kids how to shake hands. Seems silly. But it's a puzzle, right? You want this piece to fit in here. You want to hold their hand. You want to explain to them that it should be firm without hurting the other person, and that you should shake hands long enough so that you're looking at someone's eyes, and that you can tell your mom or dad afterwards what color their iris was because that's good eye contact. Then you're going to practice "you" questions because everyone likes to talk about themselves. So, David, where did you go to college? Where do you live? Or David, do you have children? …. You have to teach kids that conversations are like a tennis match. The ball has to keep going over the net, and not every child knows how to do that, and so those are social skills that you can best learn at the family dinner table.

I would also suggest that you should practice gratitude.

You don't have to be religious to practice gratitude. But considering how much pressure kids have academically today, then it would make sense that either it's Friday night before the weekend starts, or it's Sunday when the weekend is ending, and it doesn't have to be a fancy meal. But let's go around the table, and let's talk about why we were lucky and why we are happy this week.[105]

• • •

Talking with Dr. Harold really was a strong reminder that we must do better by our kids when it comes to identifying and helping them with their mental health—and teaching them the skills they need to recharge. I also try to avoid phones at bedtime, the dinner table, and whenever we have family time. I'm trying to spend twenty minutes a night just asking my older daughter about her day and giving her space to reflect on whatever is on her mind. For me, these conversations have become the most important ones of my own day and I looked forward to them.

---

[105] Generally what Dr. Koplewicz shared during our conversation is factual, though to enhance the credibility of his claims, the CDC reports that the suicide rate of children aged ten to fourteen tripled from 2007 through 2018, and a peer-reviewed *JAMA* study found that since 2008, ER visits for suicidal youth increased by 5.7 percent every year. A French study on public health postpandemic found that since January 2021, there has been a significant increase in suicide attempts among teenage girls in particular. It is true that the American Academy of Pediatrics declared a national state of emergency in child and adolescent mental health in 2021. The aggregate evidence from available research underscores an increasing acknowledgment within the healthcare community—particularly the AAP—of mental health disorders as critical concerns in pediatric populations, aligning with Dr. Koplewicz's claim about mental health surpassing infectious diseases as the principal illness among children and adolescents. Sources: Sally C. Curtin and Matthew F. Garnett, "Suicide and Homicide Death Rates among Youth and Young Adults Aged 10–24: United States, 2001–2021," National Center for Health Statistics Data Brief No. 471, June 2023, https://www.cdc.gov/nchs/products/databriefs/db471.htm; Melissa C. Mercado et al., "Trends in Emergency Department Visits for Nonfatal Self-inflicted Injuries Among Youth Aged 10 to 24 Years in the United States, 2001–2015," *JAMA* 318, no. 19 (2017):1931–1933, doi:10.1001/jama.2017.13317; F. Jollant, "Suicide Prevention in France Put to the Test by COVID-19," *European Journal of Public Health* 32, no. 3 (October 2022); https://doi.org/10.1093/eurpub/ckac129.528; American Academy of Pediatrics, "AAP-AACAP-CHA Declaration of a National Emergency in Child and Adolescent Mental Health," October 19, 2021, https://www.aap.org/en/advocacy/child-and-adolescent-healthy-mental-development/aap-aacap-cha-declaration-of-a-national-emergency-in-child-and-adolescent-mental-health/.

The Journey

The Conversation Continues

> What mental health needs is more sunlight, more candor, and more unashamed conversation.
>
> **—Glenn Close**

We each carry within us all the versions of ourselves. From my childhood to NYU, to the world of Wall Street, to my time in the early days of the internet to founding companies, to husband and parent, and all the choices and decisions and experiences that make me who I am. You have all the versions of you inside as well. Hopefully, as we go through life, we learn and grow.

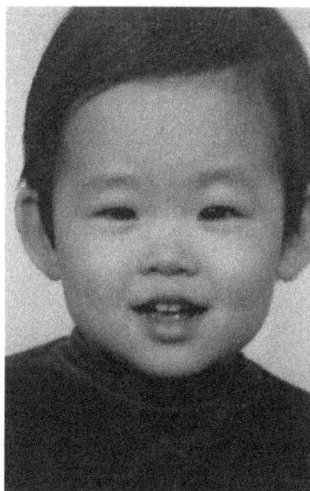

Young David Ko, circa 1973

I'd love to go back and talk to that kid—me—the one who panicked over every grade and test, who felt so much anxiety. I'd tell him, "You don't know this yet, but it's not about powering through, kid. It's about powering up."

And what I have learned is powering up means opening up and having conversations about stress and coping, and how to recharge and take care of our mental health, our internal batteries. I'd tell that kid to get out of his comfort zone, and that he could do it. I know that this book took me out of mine—and the rich rewards of talking with rebels, a rapper, and innovators have given me so much to think about as I, with intention, continue to raise the topic of recharging.

It is my hope that this book has encouraged you to check your internal battery whenever you check your phone battery. I hope you have conversations with those you love and care about, or those you lead at work, on how they are doing. Not the "You good?" variety, but with space and grace to truly listen. And then it is my hope that you encourage those you have conversations with to continue their conversation with others.

Maybe then we can heal, inspire, lead, and love, one conversation at a time. My battery, right now, is at 100%.

Recharging Our Batteries

A Guide to Mental Health Resources

Throughout this book, we've talked about the importance of recharging our mental batteries. But sometimes, we need a little extra help to plug into the right power source. That's where these resources come in.

The organizations listed here are like different types of chargers for our mental health. Some offer crisis support when our batteries are critically low. Others provide ongoing power to help maintain our charges. And some are specialized for specific mental health challenges we might face. Whether you're looking for information, support groups, or professional help, you'll find something here to assist you on your mental health journey.

Remember, reaching out for help isn't a sign of weakness—it's a powerful step toward recharging your battery and taking control of your mental health. Don't hesitate to use these resources. They're here for you, just like this book is.

Let's keep the conversation going and continue supporting each other in maintaining our mental health. After all, we're all in this together, working toward a world where everyone's battery stays fully charged.

National Alliance on Mental Illness (NAMI)

https://www.nami.org/support-education/nami-helpline/

Provides education, support, and advocacy for individuals and families affected by mental illness.

If you are struggling with your mental health, the NAMI HelpLine is here for you. Connect with a NAMI HelpLine volunteer today. Call 1 (800) 950-NAMI (6264), available Monday through Friday, 10:00 a.m. to 10:00 p.m. ET. Or text "HelpLine" to 62640, or email helpline@nami.org.

Substance Abuse and Mental Health Services Administration (SAMHSA)

1 (800) 662-HELP (4357); https://www.samhsa.gov/

SAMHSA's National Helpline is a free, confidential, 24/7, 365-day-a-year treatment referral and information service (in English and Spanish) for individuals and families facing mental and/or substance use disorders.

American Foundation for Suicide Prevention

https://afsp.org/; call or text 988 or text TALK to 741741

Provides crisis support and resources for suicide prevention.

Anxiety and Depression Association of America (ADAA)

https://adaa.org/

Offers information and support for anxiety, depression, and related disorders.

National Eating Disorders Association (NEDA)

https://www.nationaleatingdisorders.org/; crisis text line: "HOME" to 741-741

Provides support and resources for individuals and families affected by eating disorders.

The Trevor Project

https://www.thetrevorproject.org/; text "START" to 678-678, or call at 1 (866) 488-7386, or go online to chat.

Offers crisis intervention and suicide prevention services for LGBTQ+ youth. Connect to a crisis counselor 24/7, 365 days a year, from anywhere in the United States. The Trevor Project is 100 percent confidential and 100 percent free.

Mental Health America

https://mhanational.org/

Provides screening tools, educational resources, and advocacy for mental health.

Alcoholics Anonymous (AA) and Narcotics Anonymous (NA)

https://www.aa.org/; https://www.narcotics.com/

Support groups for individuals recovering from substance use disorders.

RAINN (Rape, Abuse & Incest National Network)

https://rainn.org/; call at (800) 656-HOPE, or chat online at online. rainn.org (chat en Español: rainn.org/es)

The nation's largest anti-sexual-violence organization carrying out programs to prevent sexual violence, help survivors, and ensure that perpetrators are brought to justice.

Postpartum Support International

https://www.postpartum.net/; call the PSI HelpLine at 1 (800) 944-4773, or text "Help" to (800) 944-4773 (en Español: 971-203-7773).

Offers resources and support for perinatal mood and anxiety disorders.

National Center for PTSD

https://www.ptsd.va.gov/; PTSD information voicemail: (802) 296-6300

Provides information and resources for those dealing with post-traumatic stress disorder.

Child Mind Institute

https://childmind.org/; to make an appointment, call (212) 308-3118 or request an appointment online at https://childmind.org/care/request-appointment/.

Offers resources and support for children's mental health issues.

American Sleep Association

https://aasm.org/

Provides information and resources for sleep disorders.

International OCD Foundation

https://iocdf.org/

Offers support and resources for obsessive-compulsive disorder.

Depression and Bipolar Support Alliance

https://www.dbsalliance.org/

Provides in-person and online support groups give people living with depression and bipolar disorder a safe, welcoming place to share experiences, discuss coping skills, and offer each other hope.

National Alliance for Caregiving

https://www.caregiving.org/

Offers resources and support for caregivers of individuals with mental health conditions.

The Calm Blog

https://www.calm.com/blog

In tandem with the Calm app, our clinically backed articles and resources on the Calm blog are here to help you stress less, sleep more, live mindfully, and feel better, wherever you are on your mental health journey.

Rayze

Founded by NFL veteran Carl Nassib, Rayze is a mobile platform that transforms philanthropy by using social media to streamline giving back. It connects users with volunteer opportunities, facilitates easy donations, and fosters a community focused on authentic, uplifting content. https://rayzeapp.com/

How to Breast Cancer

How to Breast Cancer founded by Amelia O'Relly offers a streamlined, user-friendly platform to guide individuals through their breast cancer journey. It provides essential tools, information, and support for patients, caregivers, and loved ones, all in one place. https://www.thebreastcancerguide.com/

The 5 Resets

Dr. Aditi Nerurkar presents a revolutionary approach to tackling stress and burnout in her book *The 5 Resets*. With over twenty years of clinical experience, she offers practical, science-backed strategies for lasting resilience.

Center for Humane Technology (CHT)

To learn more about CHT's work and access resources and toolkits, visit https://www.humanetech.com.

www.ingramcontent.com/pod-product-compliance
Lightning Source LLC
Chambersburg PA
CBHW031536260326
41914CB00032B/1834/J

* 9 7 9 8 8 8 7 5 0 4 9 4 0 *